Ethics, Management and Mythology

Rational decision making for health service professionals

Michael Loughlin

Lecturer in Philosophy and
Professional Ethics and Critical Thinking
Manchester Metropolitan University

Foreword by

David Seedhouse

RADCLIFFE MEDICAL PRESS

Radcliffe Medical Press Ltd
18 Marcham Road, Abingdon, Oxon OX14 1AA, United Kingdom

www.radcliffe-oxford.com
The Radcliffe Medical Press electronic catalogue and online ordering
facility.
Direct sales to anywhere in the world.

British Library Cataloguing in Publication Data

A catalogue record for this book is available from the British Library.

ISBN 1 85775 574 X

Typeset by Joshua Associates Ltd, Oxford
Printed and bound by TJ International Ltd, Padstow, Cornwall

Contents

Foreword

Michael Loughlin writes so that we might see ourselves without illusion and without excuse for the banalities and barbarities we inflict on each other. We flatter ourselves that we are civilised yet we habitually place conformity before reason, tragically forgetting that without thought, morality is nothing.

How, he asks, can we stop ourselves being so bloody stupid?

Loughlin's primary study is the denial of reason in health service management. Health services have always been managed one way or another: by doctors individually and in private companies, by public bodies and – in Britain since the mid-1980s – by designated health managers determined to establish themselves as a profession.

Partly to separate themselves from other healthcare tribes, health managers invented their own vocabulary. They talk of 'total quality', 'health output', 'case mix', 'management-led initiatives', 'DRGs' and 'QALYs' as if these generalisations are as concrete as the bottom line of a commercial balance sheet. But nobody, however influential, can create reality from jargon, however often they spout it.

Health managers say they need an ethical code because it is important for a profession to have ethical standards. But having standards is quite different from thinking carefully about what one is doing. Codes foster the self-satisfied view that 'So long as I obey this principle my practice will be within ethical conventions', when what is really required is a perpetual questioning of circumstance and self: How did this troublesome situation arise? How can I achieve the most moral solution? What do I mean by 'most moral solution'?

Most ethical difficulties in health services – resource allocation, truth telling, balancing medical and social priorities – are generated by the set-up of health services themselves. Consequently, adhering to codes created from within cannot possibly produce better ethical systems (imagine a slave owners' code of ethics and the point is obvious).

The answer to Loughlin's question is not yet another professional code.

> '. . . we [do not] solve the real ethical problems generated by our practices by constructing a "professional ethic" and simply asserting that the problems are now solved. Instead, we need to find ways to educate ourselves: we need to develop methods of reasoning and methods of coping which will equip us to deal effectively with the problems we face in real contexts.'

We must look at ourselves and we must learn to 'do philosophy', not as the professionals define it (as an exclusive, elitist activity that only supposedly very clever people can do) but as an everyday activity, a remedy for the smog of idiocy that constantly threatens to overwhelm us.

Unfortunately, not only do defenders of the 'new management thinking' shy away from serious reflection about health management, they don't want anyone else doing it either. When confronted with reasoned criticisms from anyone not part of their 'unique management culture', their attitude is: We have specialist knowledge, techniques and standards. Since you are not one of us, you cannot understand these as we do, so there is no point in our listening to you. Which explains their constant references to their special insights, their 'unique leadership paradigm' and 'distinctively managerial perspective'. Their faith in these totems is so complete that some of them claim that managers should not have to defend their views by means of what others regard as 'the processes of rational thought'. Loughlin finds this attitude repugnant, which is why he reacts with such outrage against management-speak and the foolish postmodern claim that racist butchers are no less moral than voluntary aid workers.

His book is the perfect antidote for empty-headed relativism. Read it and you are bound to agree that the managers' escape clause is nonsense. Whatever your culture, there is reason and there is logic and these truths apply throughout the world so far as anyone can understand it.

Like Orwell, Loughlin urges us to take courage in the face of our collective psychosis.

> 'To lack any rational intuitions is to have lost the ability to distinguish sense from nonsense, to have become as intellectually and emotionally pliable as a model citizen of Orwell's Oceania (a spin-doctor's ideal society).'

Winston's job at the Ministry of Truth (in Orwell's *1984*) was to rewrite history, a job he found fundamentally distressing.

> 'The past not only changed, but changed continuously. What most afflicted him with the sense of nightmare was that he had never clearly understood why the huge imposture was undertaken. The immediate advantages of falsifying the past were obvious, but the ultimate motive was more mysterious. He took up his pen and wrote:
>
> I understand HOW: I do not understand WHY . . .
>
> In the end the Party would announce that two and two made five, and you would have to believe it. It was inevitable that they should make the claim sooner or later: the logic of their position demanded it. Not merely the validity of experience, but the very existence of external reality, was tacitly denied by their philosophy. The heresy of heresies was common sense.'

Deciding not to think is a natural human reaction to existential threat. It is terrifying to have only one intellect, one personal experience of pain, one inevitable and solitary death. So we hurl ourselves at other people, trying to bury ourselves deep within their customs. To belong, to forget, to ease the pain.

Part of our nature compels us to wear the daub and head-dress of the tribe (any will do, so long as we are anaesthetised). But we do not have to succumb. We are equipped with brains that can easily overcome our need to hide, if only we can find the courage to think for ourselves.

So Michael Loughlin's book is a call to arms. It is a guide to the reclamation of intelligence and the restoration of pride in doing the right thing as we perceive it, not as we are told to perceive it. It is an ancient message. And yet it is one that must be restated throughout the ages, by fresh writers opposed to the debilitating dumbness to which we so often submit.

It might be said that Loughlin is big on objections and short on solutions. Not only is this a misunderstanding of his philosophical position, it is to fail to see its practicality. It is foolish for anyone, never mind a philosopher advocating a case for independent thought, to specify how others should live. But nevertheless, it is possible to say what a philosophically aware health services manager should be. For Loughlin, he or she should:

- not accept his social and working environment as necessary
- be open to the possibility that he is mistaken, even fundamentally
- be self-critical
- understand how little he knows
- be continually willing to think about what words mean and imply
- continually reflect on what it is wise and moral to do
- continually reflect on where to draw the line – to work out when not to accept a situation or policy as given, despite tradition
- be continually willing to develop political strategies to resolve difficult situations
- reason logically.

As you study this list, you will note that the manager described is hardly typical of our present crop; rather, he is philosophical in the central sense of the term. But you should also notice that Loughlin's manager is not impractical. Indeed, once he decides to make a difference he must be deeply pragmatic, his clarity of thought will naturally lead to a clarity of purpose and outcome.

He will, for instance, realise the hopelessness of trying to come up with a morally sound rationing scheme, since this is impossible for conceptual reasons that can be easily understood (having read Loughlin). But he might decide instead to initiate an education programme in moral reasoning for clinicians and managers. His philosophical skills would tell him that the first project is impractical whereas the second (which to many will sound irrelevant) is both central to the problems he encounters every day and is a potential solution to some of them (since its aim would be to free its students' intellects from their existential dread).

This book won't change the world but, like all examples of the higher human faculties used with passion and insight, it will be a catalyst for change in some readers' lives. Read it and it is possible to see the social world stripped bare of convention and posturing, to learn to see it for what it really is. And once you can do that you can at least decide for yourself what you make of it.

David Seedhouse BA PhD
Professor of Health and Social Ethics,
Auckland University of Technology, New Zealand,
and Professor of Healthcare Analysis,
Middlesex University, UK
August 2001

Introduction

This book is about critical thinking. Although aimed primarily at health services management, it is in fact for anyone who wants to think critically about their working practices and the general conduct of their lives. It is a work of 'ethics' in the proper sense of the word and, as such, its scope is not meant to be limited to its main target audience. This much is made obvious in the opening comments.

The views expressed about management theory and bioethics are already known to some of the exponents of these approaches to organisation and ethics, since I have published several articles on these topics. Since my arguments and conclusions have been subject to (sometimes wilful) misinterpretation in the past, I have no doubt that they will be again, but since it is always worth trying to spell things out as clearly as possible there are a couple of points worth making right at the beginning.

In Part Two of this work I look at contemporary management theory and I conclude that most of it is conceptually flawed, jargon riddled and even dangerous. It is, as we academics are wont to put it, a load of old tosh.

In Part Three I look at what bioethicists have had to say about the ethics of health services management and I conclude firstly that it is a mistake to try to solve the problems in this area by constructing a discipline called 'the ethics of health services management' (indeed, that the project is impossible) and secondly that some of the problems of health services organisation cannot be solved within the current social context of the service, such that a responsible decision maker will recognise the inevitable arbitrariness of the 'solutions' offered to these problems. (I go on to say that one of the key goals of moral education must be to enable us to find ways to cope with such situations, to identify their causes and to develop adequate responses to them.)

The defenders of these theoretical approaches have chosen to interpret these points as meaning that I think that anyone who works in health services organisation is incapable of thinking rationally or morally about any issue. Instead of responding to my arguments (which in general they have not even attempted to understand) they have elected to construe my detailed criticisms of their own favoured theories as an attack on an entire group of workers in the health service and have condemned me on these grounds. A simple analogy should help to dispel this rather stupid and unwarranted reading of my position.

It is my view that much of what passes for 'education theory' is also nonsense and I do not think that there is any such thing as the discipline 'the ethics of educators'. Does it follow from this that I think that all educators are in fact stupid people or that it is impossible to think intelligently or ethically about educational practices? This would be a bizarre position for someone who works as a teacher to take. Rather, my view is that we do not need teachers who are well versed in the most fashionable 'education' jargon, nor do we solve the real ethical problems of our practices by constructing a 'professional ethic' and simply asserting that the problems are now solved. Instead, we need to find ways to educate *ourselves*: we need to develop methods of reasoning and methods of coping which will equip us to deal effectively with the problems we face in real contexts. We need to think of ourselves primarily not as teachers, managers or whatever, but as intelligent human beings who happen to occupy specific social roles and we need to be aware of the social context which circumscribes those roles and the limits it places upon us. We cannot simply take the moral significance of these roles for granted in our moral thinking about them.

Similar points are explained and defended in some detail in the text, with specific reference to health services management. The public services need people with well-developed thinking skills, not people who can recite trendy jargon. We do not help managers to think intelligently about their role by filling their heads with rubbish. We certainly don't help them by forcing them to learn this rubbish in order to 'qualify' as 'management specialists' and then to implement it against the wishes of the workforce. If we do decide to help managers 'find a role for themselves' in this way, then the role they find will be neither a useful nor a very popular one in the context of the service where they must spend their working lives.

Since some of the arguments in support of these claims are complex, I have incorporated an analytical table of contents, which goes through the entire book in some detail, attempting a précis of the main points under each subheading. This is not meant to be read instead of the book. Rather, it is an attempt to make its logical structure explicit so that, if the reader should get lost at any point along the way she may turn to it for guidance and regain her sense of the overall direction. Analytical tables are a common feature of older philosophy books and they seem to me to be one of many currently unfashionable ideas well worth reviving.

Analytical table
of contents

Chapter 1

3–6: This book is about acquiring the skill of sustained, systematic critical thinking. If you are looking for a quick fix for some very specific set of problems then this book is not for you. Rather, it aims to affect the way in which you approach practical problems, providing a vantage point from which a range of problems may be fruitfully considered and a method of reasoning applicable not only to the problems discussed in these pages but also to new problems which may emerge in the context of the reader's own practice.

6–15: Most books about management and ethics contain case studies. These are useful aids to decision making only if used to elucidate the underlying processes of reasoning at work in their analysis. We need to ask: what does it mean to be a 'good' decision maker? What sort of individuals do we want making decisions and what kinds of processes are likely to produce that sort of person? Each one of us can ask: how do I become that sort of person?

15–21: Philosophical analysis (sometimes called 'conceptual analysis') is a method of reasoning which enables us to examine the conceptual maps which underlie practical thinking. Good decision making requires the exercise of sound intuition and this requires in the background a sophisticated conceptual map. These 'maps' represent ways in which experiences may be organised and they embody assumptions, which may be true or false. The goal of philosophical analysis therefore is to liberate practical thinking from the influence of false assumptions and theories which may inhibit good decision making.

21–26: The book is structured in such a way that it enables the reader to build up an adequate map of the territory to be negotiated. In the process of building this map something happens to you: you become someone who systematically reflects on practical problems, someone who thinks clearly, who can recognise dogma and sophistry and expose it for what it is, who can look at the world from new angles until she finds the right perspective.

Chapter 2

27–31: Some authors claim that 'ethics' refers to public, legalistic 'codes of practice' while 'morality' refers to something personal, private and subjective. While it is possible to employ the words in this way, the utility of this usage can be questioned. Codes of practice have a role in rational decision making but rational thinking cannot be reduced to following rules. A more helpful and intellectually defensible distinction is as follows. 'Ethics' is the systematic study of morality and morality concerns the way we live our lives, the choices we make, the sort of people we are. To ask moral questions is to ask questions about how to live and practise: it is to search for good reasons for the way one behaves.

31–38: To search for reasons is to seek to practise rationally. Theories of ethics are therefore theories of rational decision making. The egoist says that rationality means 'self-interest' but on close examination it is not clear what this means or why we should believe it. Postmodernism questions the possibility of rationality, claiming that the ideas of 'reason' and 'truth' have been rendered suspect. Although such claims are fashionable in certain academic circles, their intellectual defence and practical implications are unclear and they seem ultimately to be self-defeating.

38–44: An ethical subjectivist claims that it is impossible to establish the truth of any value judgement by rational means: only factual judgements can really be true. While there are serious questions about what counts as 'evidence' for the claim that we should do one thing rather than another, all thinking (about 'facts' and 'values') requires the exercise of sound judgement and so implies the need for reasons. Ethical theories concern what counts as a good reason to behave in one way rather than another and how we can know this.

44–54: Consequentialist moral theory explains what we have reason to do in terms of whatever action brings about the best overall consequences in the situation which faces us. The most famous variant of consequentialism is utilitarianism. Deontologists claim that there are non-consequential reasons for action, including responsibilities generated by personal commitments and absolute or unconditional duties we allegedly have to all other persons, duties which present themselves (to the consciousness of the responsible moral agent) as inviolable rules. These 'rules' are sometimes claimed to reflect the basic rights of persons. Nozick refers to them as 'side-constraints' upon action. An attempted compromise position is called 'rule utilitarianism'.

54–60: The theories help us to identify the different types of concern at work in moral thinking, but they provide no basis to decide between these different types of concern in cases where they conflict. Furthermore, they do not explain adequately how we know which concerns are relevant in any given situation. More serious critical attention needs to be given to the faculty of intuition. Unfortunately, the most famous attempts to explain intuition resort to mysticism and seem beset by logical problems and fallacies.

Chapter 3

63–67: For some years now, much of the work in management theory has been devoted to the construction of a new and rather strange language to describe and evaluate practice. This language originates in the world of business but its use has spread to the public services and its terminology increasingly infiltrates political conversation. Its exponents seek to make it the adoptive mother tongue in every area of professional life but they are meeting with resistance and there are ideological underpinnings to the struggle.

67–73: A distinctive feature of this language is its use of the word 'quality'. There are management 'philosophies', approaches or 'paradigms' called Total Quality Management, Continuous Quality Improvement and even Industrial Quality Management Science. These approaches are employed but their conceptual foundations remain unexplained, shrouded in baffling jargon. At no point is 'quality' defined, nor is it explained how it can be the object of scientific study or 'engineered': these assumptions appear to be articles of faith.

73–76: The only substance to the concept of 'quality' seems to be that certain people are prepared to say that a thing has quality. This gives us a clue as to the real meaning of 'quality science'. What is happening is 'persuasive definition': by continually describing certain products or practices as 'demonstrating quality' it is possible to create an atmosphere in which it seems unreasonable to question or criticise the dominant policies and ethos. The purpose of the 'quality revolution' is the manipulation of opinions.

Chapter 4

77–80: Management theorists sometimes claim that there are 'basic organisational criteria' common to all complex organisations. By 'incorporating' these 'criteria' (sometimes also called 'principles') into health and other 'service industries', practices will necessarily be improved. However, the 'criteria' are not explained in detail: rather, they are spelled out in terms so abstract and general as to be platitudinous and managers are given no clear guidance as to how to apply them in practice.

80–87: As a result, policy documents produced by management and government organisations are increasingly composed almost entirely of slogans and buzzwords, with little in the way of substance and clarity. The vacuous nature of such material can be explained with reference to the intellectual bankruptcy of its underlying assumptions. Management is not a 'science' in the sense that engineering is: what it means for a building to stand up does not change in accordance with the purposes for which it is used but what it means for an organisation to be 'successful' does.

87–89: The attempt to apply principles of good organisation derived from one context (business) to a radically different one (the health service) represents a philosophical error. There are no principles of good organisational practice that (i) are generally applicable and (ii) have any substantial implications. Instead of recognising this error, management theorists treat objections to their theories as evidence of ignorance or psychological disorder on the part of objectors, who need to be 'enlightened'. There are three reasons for their confidence.

89–91: Firstly, the sheer volume of the work in the area seems to some theorists to be an argument in itself. But the very fact that an idea is fashionable and has the backing of the powers that be does not prove it is correct.

91–98: Secondly, many authors are confused by the grammatical properties of the word 'quality', which they treat as a referring expression. Logical confusions such as this can lead to mystification: hence the strange, quasi-religious tone of some of the literature in the area.

98–104: The third reason concerns the influence of ideology. To grasp the benefits of the new management thinking, we are required to construe health as a 'product' and to regard the process of caring as a 'production process', governed by the same 'basic principles' and 'values' as any commercial venture. Carers must come to see the patient as a 'customer' or 'consumer'. Managers are encouraged to be 'leaders' in a social project which aims to make every aspect of professional (and eventually social) life comprehensible in terms of the same free market ideology.

105–113: It is not clear that managers should want to take on this role, nor is it necessary that they do so. The social project in question is destructive to the values and purposes of healthcare, education and the public service ethos. Management organisations should take the lead in broadening the debate, instead of condoning the destruction in the name of 'pragmatism'. We need to ask fundamental questions about what sort of a society we want and how it can provide the services we need. We need to foster an atmosphere of critical discussion of all the assumptions that frame the current debate about healthcare.

Chapter 5

117–119: A society where philosophy is deemed irrelevant to practical concerns is a society unable to analyse its most fundamental assumptions and, as such, is an ideologue's paradise. It is no coincidence that the decline in the fortunes of philosophy has been accompanied by a rise in the influence and status of the political 'spin doctor', whose science is the manipulation of an intellectually disempowered populace.

119–126: The decline of philosophy and the current misconceptions surrounding the subject are, at least in part, the product of a doctrine promoted enthusiastically by philosophers themselves for much of the 20th century. Although today it is widely held that logical empiricism (or positivism) is false, its assumptions still influence political conversation and even the work of applied philosophers.

126–128: It would therefore be a mistake to write off logical positivism, and the irrationalist view of ethics it gives rise to, without attempting to understand its influence and appeal. There is much that needs to be preserved in its critique of certain views which may be labelled 'rationalist'. We need, then, to understand its appeal when constructing an account of practical decision making which can incorporate the role of rationality and intuition and so represent an advance on the theories already considered.

128–132: Irrationalism provides a good description of moral and political discourse in contemporary liberal societies. However, the fact that public debate frequently conforms to the irrationalist picture does not show that this is how it must be or should be. Rather, it betrays the intellectual poverty of contemporary political conversation.

132–137: An adequate account of moral psychology explains the relationship between 'feelings' and 'reasoning' and provides the basis for a better form of ethical intuitionism than the form considered in Chapter 2. Intuitions may be construed as rational dispositions and the main reason for embracing the discipline of philosophy is to develop and sustain the right sort of dispositions in ourselves and others. We might call this view philosophy as training in intellectual and moral self-defence.

Chapter 6

139–143: Unfortunately, many applied philosophers reject this view of the subject. In their view, for philosophy to be properly 'practical' it must produce 'principles, goals or guidelines' for the ethical running of the health service. This view reflects a division between 'theory' and 'practice' which suggests that the role of theorists is to produce sets of rules for practitioners to follow. This mentality is at work in some of the statements made by defenders of the National Institute for Clinical Excellence (NICE). It is the wrong view of the theory–practice relationship and risks turning practitioners of all sorts into uncritical rule followers.

143–146: The distinction between 'pure' and 'applied' philosophy is unhelpful and reflects a simplistic view of what it means to 'apply' any theoretical approach to practice. Philosophy is valuable primarily as a method of analysis. It can only be of any real use to people if it enables them to understand the true nature and causes of the problems which confront them.

146–150: To do this properly it must require them to think honestly and critically about the roles they occupy and the forces and structures which shape those roles. Forms of 'applied ethics' which do not do this are practically useless and intellectually unsatisfactory. They may even serve to confuse and mislead, so actually inhibiting moral and intellectual progress.

150–155: That branch of philosophy which attempts to apply ethical theory to the problems of the health service (including health services management) is often called 'bioethics'. For bioethics to avoid being a positively harmful subject, its exponents must think very carefully about the irrational nature of the context they hope to affect and the limits this places upon their enterprise. They must ask the question: 'Who is my audience?'

155–158: The goal of the 'rationing debate' within bioethics is not to reduce the suffering of 'de-prioritised' patients, but to find a theoretical rationale for that suffering or for some specific distribution of suffering. Despite the honourable intent of some of its participants, this debate is, in an important sense, misguided.

158–162: Success in bioethics often means producing 'positive' conclusions, meaning solutions which work given the system as it is. Thus 'the system works' acquires by default the status of a fundamental truth. This discourages individuals working within the system from critically examining fundamental assumptions.

162–168: The intellectual character of the rationing debate is shaped and limited by certain assumptions of market economics, the key one being the economic assumption of 'scarcity'. The problem with economic solutions is that they encourage us to ignore both the incommensurability of certain values and the broader social context which gives rise to the problems under discussion. They therefore risk providing rationalisations for policies rather than ethically sound defences of policies.

168–170: It is easy to justify decisions with reference to principles spelled out in such vague terms that almost anyone could accept them. The trouble is, such principles could justify different and incompatible answers to the same practical questions – so they don't provide any real practical guidance.

171–176: Similar problems beset the quality-adjusted life year (QALY). Different methods of aggregation can provide different answers to questions about what policy produces the most QALYs and there is no way of knowing which is the 'right' method.

176–182: The presence of moral philosophers on 'ethical committees' fails (by the admission of these philosophers) to bring the methods of philosophy into the policy making process. Their presence helps to foster the illusion that decisions of state are the result of impartial, objective reasoning 'informed' by 'experts'. They bestow academic credibility on policies and on the whole policy-forming procedure, making it subsequently harder for others, particularly those lacking academic standing, to criticise the policies.

form of relativism called 'conventionalism'. Though unsatisfactory, subjectivism is more consistent than conventionalism. The latter arbitrarily privileges the practices of groups of people over individuals, requiring no rational justification for entrenched group preferences.

216–221: The only consistent alternative to subjectivism is moral realism. Our ability to criticise the conventions underlying whole ways of life is fundamental to our common-sense conception of moral thinking. If a theory causes us to deny the most obvious features of rational life, we have grounds to search for a better theory – one that is able to make sense of them. Moral realism succeeds in this respect where subjectivism and conventionalism fail.

221–230: Moral realism also provides the basis for an approach to moral education which incorporates the advantages of the two approaches already discussed, while avoiding their respective pitfalls. It is possible to reconcile the values of 'individuality' and 'community', 'autonomy' and 'the good life' via a relational account of what it is to be human.

Chapter 8

231–233: The key virtues necessary to manage well are 'self-direction' and 'solidarity' and the most important skill is that of balancing the exercise of these virtues with the need to survive in the context of an often irrational professional environment. This is the problem of preserving one's integrity.

233–236: To do this it is essential to develop a sound intuitive grasp of the distinction between social realism and moral realism and the relationship between the two. This distinction is important since without it we cannot have a proper appreciation of the difference between thinking about moral starting points and thinking about tactics.

236–244: At the moment management education, along with vocational education generally, seems to be heading in quite the wrong direction. If vocational education is to be a good thing, then it must represent a partnership between the academic and the practical. Instead, it creates artificial divisions between the two and as a result is neither one thing nor the other: neither properly practical nor properly academic. The most important component of moral education is the capacity for emotional identification. A mistaken idea of 'objectivity' has for too long influenced thinking about moral education in general and the education of managers in particular.

244–247: Management organisations could do a lot more to create environments in which good practice can flourish. Instead, they often help to create environments which breed cynicism and cowardice. It is important that managers, and their organisations, are able to identify and criticise nonsense and to reconsider their moral relationships with their fellow workers and society as a whole. This is not where the debate should end: rather, it is where the sensible debate should begin.

Part One

Management, morals and philosophy: a start

Chapter 1

Who this book is for and who it is not for[1]

There are already too many books offering solutions to the problems of the health service. Scattered across the libraries and bookshops of the civilised world, whole forests lie dead in the shape of texts and journal articles, discussing such subjects as the solution of 'ethical dilemmas' in health services management and the development of just and practicable policies for the future organisation of healthcare. This book is a little different. It does discuss health service organisation and policy and it is a work of theory but, unlike much of the literature purporting to 'apply' theory to practice, this book makes no attempt to present the reader with a set of neat solutions to the real and complex ethical problems it examines. Nor, like so much of the work in this area, does it present a set of untidy solutions to a series of artificial or oversimplified problems. Indeed, it is one of its central claims that, in the sense meant by most of the authors in the field, a 'solution' to the problems of health services organisation is rendered impossible by the social and political context in which the health service must function (*see* Chapter 6).

Instead, this work offers the reader a starting point, a place to begin thinking seriously about health services management and policy. Read it carefully and without preconception and the book should alter not your views on some specific question or set of questions but the *way* in which you think about *any* practical question. If successful, the book will enable the reader to acquire a vantage point from which a whole range of problems may fruitfully be considered and a method of reasoning applicable not only to the problems discussed in these pages, but also to new problems which may emerge in the context of the reader's own practice.

More will be said about the philosophical method of reasoning which the book both promotes and exemplifies and whose propagation was my ulterior motive when I began writing articles on health services management some years ago. (*See*, in particular, Chapter 5 but also the discussion of moral education in Part Four.) For now, it is worth noting the sheer immodesty of the claim being made here. Some books, like the TV repair manual, keep a respectable distance from the reader throughout: they present a description of some problems followed by a set of steps the reader can go through, should she ever feel the need, to solve those problems. Having read the book, she can then go on with her life as before, totally unchanged as a person, seeing the world in the same way as before; she may have acquired some new items of knowledge but what she *is*, her attitudes, her basic assumptions about the world and her *style* of thinking – these things remain fundamentally unaffected and unchallenged by the experience of reading the book.

No serious academic book, and certainly no work of philosophy, can be like that since philosophy, unlike a repair manual, cannot aim to limit its significance to a narrow range of possibilities. The issues it deals with are too important, too fundamental and too pervasive in nature for it to be possible to address them sensibly without 'interfering' with the reader's picture of her life and practice. Printed in bold on the front cover of my copy of Robert Pirsig's *Zen and the Art of Motorcycle Maintenance* are the words 'THIS BOOK WILL CHANGE THE WAY YOU FEEL AND THINK ABOUT YOUR LIFE'. Pirsig's is a wonderful book, even though the philosophical position it expounds is founded upon a fallacy. Surprisingly, a great deal of the so-called 'management theory' popular today is founded upon the exact same fallacy: a basic conceptual error concerning the meaning of 'quality', which will be discussed in detail later in this work (Chapter 4).

Despite this, and its unlikely connection with management theory, Pirsig's book has got it right in one important respect. Books should aim to affect their readers' lives, to change the way they think about their experience and practices. A book which attempts to do this aims to achieve something significant. It takes itself seriously and in so doing, takes its readers seriously, treating them as people whose time is not to be wasted with trivia. Books that don't even try to do this are an unconscionable waste of trees. It is a testimony to the poverty of our culture that we expect so little from books, that the claim made for Pirsig's work will seem to many to be somehow arrogant or pretentious. It shows how stupid we have become, how unused we are to intellectual exercise, how little we value our precious time and how much contempt we have acquired for the written word. This book, like Pirsig's, is not just *about* real life: it attempts to *affect* the world via its readers, by influencing the way they think about their lives. If it has the desired effect on even one person, it will be a success.

So who is this book for? If you think that a good book is one that tells you 'all you need to know' about a given subject, so that you can read it once, then never have to read or think again, then this book is not for you. This book requires you to think; it does not attempt to do your thinking for you. If you expect a properly 'practical' book to get all the problems it discusses 'sorted out', providing a checklist of dos and don'ts to be followed mechanically for a quick fix, then this book is not for you. Real life obviously isn't like that: it is never 'sorted out' and we do not even begin to live and practise well until we learn this.

This book is for you if you want to become a more thoughtful person, a more capable reasoner, a more perceptive analyst. It is for you if you are prepared to engage in rigorous and sometimes frustrating intellectual exercise in the pursuit of this goal. If you wish to skip straight to the concluding chapter then you can of course do so, but you will profit from this as much as you did when, in school, you turned straight to the back of the maths book for the answers. What you need is to do the working out. You need to go through all the stages, to get a sense of the shape and depth of the problems, to explore possible solutions, often to find that they do not work, then to come to understand why they do not work and to search for new approaches. This way you build up a picture of the territory you want to negotiate and in the process something happens to you: you become someone who systematically reflects on practical problems, someone who thinks clearly, who can recognise dogma and sophistry and expose them for what they are, who can look at the world from new angles until she finds the right perspective. You become philosophically competent. To find the way out of any 'moral maze' one must learn, first of all, what an exit would look like. This is so for the moral problems inherent in health services management and it is so for all moral problems, in any area. As we will see, once the terms are properly understood, all practical problems are really moral problems.

Thus, while this book is primarily for those with an interest in health services management and policy (which is all of us, since these issues affect the well-being of every living soul) it is, more generally, for anyone who wants to think more rigorously about their practices. It is, in short, for anyone sane enough to feel the need for clear thinking in an increasingly bizarre and confusing world. It is for anyone who hears nonsense and knows it to be nonsense but cannot quite say why, cannot explain exactly how they know. It is for anyone who does not know what philosophy is or why it is relevant to real life. It is also for philosophers who have forgotten why their discipline needs to be applied to the concerns of everyday life, if it is to take up its proper place in human affairs and to be treated with the respect it deserves.

The health service doesn't need a repair manual: to proceed as if it does is to beg all the important questions about how we should identify and conceptualise its problems in the first place. This does not claim to be the only work you should read in order to address these questions sensibly, but it is a good place to start.

A way in

We can get a clearer sense of the general approach by considering what is wrong with most other books about management and ethics. Very often such works contain 'case studies': descriptions of scenarios, real or imagined, which the reader is invited to consider, typically with a view to deciding what one or more of the characters described 'should do' about their problems. For instance:

'*Restructuring has occurred. This gives the head of section an opportunity to reallocate some members of staff to different roles. Time constraints leave little time to consult with staff. Furthermore, senior management insists that further information regarding restructuring cannot be released by heads of section until agreement has been reached. Rumours in the informal networks are rife, ranging from fear of redundancy . . . to staff being reallocated to completely different sections. The ensuing level of uncertainty results in anxiety which begins to affect work, competency and output. What should the line manager do?*' (Henry 1995, p. 105)

'*It is four weeks before a general election. The district is over-spending and the DGM wishes to advise the DHA that a local GP hospital should be closed to save money. The sitting MP, anxious about his marginal seat, accuses the DGM of "playing politics". How should the DGM react?*' (Wall 1989, p. 105)

Such cases are meant to give a 'practical' feel to the text, but for the most part this feeling is illusory. We have to ask: what precisely is the educational function of such examples? What does the reader learn that is of practical value by considering them? This depends largely on what the author goes on to say about them. For the reader is surely aware, before reading the text, that such situations exist. The point of reading a book about ethics is to develop defensible responses, not to the specific (usually made-up) cases described in the book but to a range of actual and possible problems which either have occurred, or might occur, in the reader's own experience. Thus, the study will only be of any real use if the reader learns something of a sufficiently general nature to be abstracted from the discussion of the case and applied to her own life. In some of the better applied ethics texts, such studies are analysed in terms of the main theories of rational decision making: moral theories[2] such as utilitarianism and the various forms of deontology are described and used to bring out the different types of consideration that a situation can present. (*See,* for instance, the five cases discussed in the first chapter of Callahan 1988.)

Alternatively, certain 'basic principles' might be postulated on the grounds that they are 'self-evident' or that they at least command near-universal support, and the cases discussed in terms of these principles. The problems with this particular approach are too numerous to list here, although a more detailed criticism of this whole genre of theory will be presented in Chapter 6. The basic problem is that, when spelled out to any degree of specificity, no substantial moral principle is self-evident, nor does any such principle command universal or even near-universal support. For instance, the most famous exponents of the 'principles' approach, Beauchamp and Childress (1994), effectively assume that justice is possible within a capitalist society like their own, yet there are many credible positions in political philosophy which hold that capitalism necessarily generates unacceptable social and economic inequalities and as a consequence is inherently unjust. The point is that the authors' 'four principles' command broad support only for so long as they are left so vague as to be open to numerous, and mutually incompatible, interpretations. The liberal and the socialist alike believe in justice, they only disagree about what justice really means. Similarly we might agree, verbally, that any decision made in the context of health services management should be 'fair' to all affected parties, but if our intuitions about what is actually fair differ, then we have no substantial agreement about anything. It makes little sense to say that a set of principles provides a firm foundation for decision making if, when we attempt to apply them in any real-life context, the foundations crack apart and we are left to resort to our personal intuitive reactions in any case.

Less useful still, but sadly more representative of much of the work concerned specifically with health management, are the approaches of the works from which the above-quoted cases are taken. One of the authors purports to 'examine' practical problems in terms of a 'simple ethical framework' which, he declares in the Preface, he will make 'no attempt' to defend with reference to any ethical theory (Wall 1989). He views the complete absence of serious philosophical analysis of the 'dilemmas' he discusses as an advantage of his approach, enabling him to provide 'practical assistance' of the 'down-to-earth' variety to beleaguered practitioners. The view that one can discuss ethics sensibly without doing moral philosophy is examined in Part Three of this book and we shall see that it is based on a misconception of moral philosophy and of the relationship between theory and practice. For now, suffice it to say that the author is true to the pledge of his Preface, offering no defence nor even a clear account of any of his assumptions. What is not clear is how, by making a set of unsupported and largely unexplained assertions, he is offering 'assistance' to anyone. Why should we accept his 'framework'? How do we know if we are applying it correctly? The framework is spelled out in terminology so vague that it provides no basis for a distinction between correct and incorrect applications. Again, the reader is left to resort to her own intuitions, just as she would do if she had never read the text. Could we not manage without such assistance?

Operating at an even greater distance from critical thought, the author of the other case study adopts an 'empirical' approach, conducting a survey of opinions about 'ethics and values' whose respondents are members of her own institution. This apparently led to her being 'stretched beyond the boundaries of academia into the realms of ethical reality and everyday morality within the organisational framework' (Henry 1995, from the Preface) but at no point did it cause her to subject any of the responses to a sustained critical analysis.[3] This methodology is reminiscent of the caricature of 'non-directive therapy' presented in the novel *The Dice Man* (Reinhart 1972): in order to discover what a person should do about his problems, ask him what he thinks he should do, then repeat his answer back to him. Not that the authors actually apply their avowed methodologies, flawed as they are. What is astonishing about each of the case studies cited is that they are accompanied in their respective texts by no discussion whatsoever of the specific case described. It is not clear how this constitutes a 'study', nor is it clear what the reader is supposed to learn from this. One of the authors explains that the 'studies' are 'open-ended', advising students in a 'classroom' setting to 'explore what might be done' (Wall 1989, from the Preface). This is rather like a tennis coach leaving his tutees alone with racquets and a ball and advising them to 'explore the possibilities' contained within their situation. They might make some progress, but this hardly to the credit of the tutor.

So one problem with the use of case studies in ethics text-books is the shocking lack of attention paid by authors to the processes of reasoning involved in their analysis. Indeed, some authors plainly think that simply by inventing an imaginary case they are providing 'practical assistance' or 'guidance' to the reader. Yet even when analyses are provided, even when cases are discussed with specific reference to ethical theories, there are problems with this approach. Frequently the discussion leads only to a statement of what certain theories 'would say' or 'might say' about the case, without providing the reader with any method (other than consulting her intuitions) for determining whether or not the theory is correct to say what it does. Worse still, the claim that a particular moral theory would point to any specific solution in a concrete situation is almost always false. To make such a claim is to oversimplify the process of moral reasoning and to misrepresent the role of theory in ethical analysis. Moral theories rarely have any direct or clear-cut implications for what particular people in specific situations should do. If we learn that a certain moral philosopher sub-scribes to the theory called 'utilitarianism', this does tell us something about his views on moral matters, but it is not sufficient to tell us which way (or whether) he votes, what he thinks about the issue of abortion, whether or not he eats meat or what his stance is on the rationing of health services. Unfortunately it is rather more complicated than that. Moral thinking is not a matter of finding the true theory and reading answers off it, any more than we can ascertain the truth of Newton's Theory of Motion and use it to tell us which horse will win the 2.30 at Goodwood. The actual role of moral theory in practical decision making is a complicated and certainly controversial matter. It is worthy of our sustained attention, since if we are to develop a genuinely helpful account of practical thinking we cannot ignore the role which theories play in shaping our ideas about the world and a simplistic account is probably worse than no account at all. The discussion of this issue will therefore be developed over several sections in the work that follows. But there is a further, related problem which requires attention first.

To convey anything like a realistic account of a person's actual work context would require a lot of detail – certainly much more than is provided in either of the case studies cited above. When such scenarios are debated within a classroom setting, the discussion is usually very inconclusive. Students will respond, with some justification, that they cannot really say what the person 'should do': 'it depends' on a number of factors not specified in the description of the case. More often than not, one can 'fill in' the details in an *ad hoc* fashion (the cases are usually imaginary anyway and they are only being used for the purposes of discussion) but even then students are likely to feel that there is 'something' missing and any solutions proposed have a somewhat arbitrary flavour. It may be that my students are particularly inept or it could be that there really are no right answers, such that all decisions about what we ought to do are in fact fundamentally arbitrary. (It is amazing how many tutors and authors of texts in applied ethics are willing to embrace this conclusion, or doctrines which entail it, without noticing that this renders their own work utterly pointless. No-one needs the assistance of an 'ethicist' to make an arbitrary decision: people can do that all by themselves.)

There is, however, a better explanation. Instead of drawing, from the shortcomings of an academic exercise, unwarranted conclusions about the nature of decision making in real-life contexts, we should perhaps question the adequacy of our representation of that reality. As anyone who has come back from holiday armed with a reel of camera film discovers, a photograph of a magnificent scene never captures the full magnificence of the place as one remembers it. This is not because our memories are faulty; it is not that the place isn't really magnificent after all. (Wouldn't that be a bizarre conclusion to draw?) Rather, it is because there really is nothing quite so good as actually being there. This is, presumably, why we spend our time and money going to beautiful places, when we could more easily stay at home and watch videos of cascading waterfalls instead. When you are there within the scene you are aware of all that is around the portion of it which the photograph depicts: your sense of the whole context enables you to appreciate fully what you are seeing at any one time, as does your direct encounter with the sounds and smells and atmosphere of a place as you travel through it.

Similarly, being faced with a set of alternatives within a classroom setting or while reading a text is never quite the same as facing those alternatives in a real situation. If you are the DGM (to return to the second of the 'case studies') then your knowledge of the full context of that person's life will go way beyond anything you can state in a description, even a fairly detailed one. You will know the other characters as real people, with their own specific histories, prejudices and eccentricities and not merely as labels. You will be aware of the different relationships, alliances and animosities which exist between them. Much of your awareness will be implicit, concerning factors which you do not even consider consciously and which you would certainly never think to spell out, but which may well affect your judgement in any case.

Now it may be that one's intuition about what is right in a particular case is determined, at least in part, by various features of this surrounding context, in the same way that one's perception of the magnificence of a scene is to some extent dependent upon one's awareness of the surrounding environment. It may be difficult, or even impossible, to understand fully why a particular decision was made if one is not immersed within that particular context. Any description is an abstraction, even when its author (like the author of the 'DGM' study) has many years of experience of the type of situation under discussion. It takes the skills of a great novelist to convey a real sense of a life in all its particularity, yet this is what would be needed to enable the reader to grasp those features of a context which are genuinely unique. (I suspect that even Salman Rushdie might struggle to achieve this in a mere 11 lines, the portion of its original text taken up by the longer of the two studies cited.)

This is why students with personal experience of the type of case described can usually make more sense of the case studies than others – they can 'fill in the gaps' by remembering features of the real situations they have lived through. But then it is the student's own experience and imagination doing the work, not the sketch of the scenario itself, and there is still no guarantee that they would come to the same conclusions were they actually living within the specific context described, rather than discussing that sort of situation in the context of a classroom. (The fact that the case is usually invented makes the whole thing even more indeterminate: there is not, really, any particular context nor are there any real persons to whom the 'case study' refers. They exist, purely, 'for the purposes of discussion'.)

It strikes me that this 'abstractness', this inevitable distance from and simplification of lived reality, accounts for the artificiality of the case studies. We cannot say with any confidence what the made-up people should do, not because decision making as such is an arbitrary matter but because we invariably have insufficient information to form the basis of a meaningful discussion. That is not to say that sometimes, perhaps even frequently, there really is no right answer, nor even any answer that one can, in good conscience, describe as 'adequate'. (I will argue later that this may very often be the case. *See*, in particular, Chapter 6.) The point is that, even in such a case, one might come to understand this, and to start to think about how one should react to this realisation, only by being immersed in the context. A formal characterisation of the problem might suggest certain solutions as both possible and desirable when someone in touch with the full murky reality would instinctively, and rightly, discount them as unworkable.[4]

So what follows from this? Does it mean that theory is useless, that we should give up on rational analysis and leave it to individuals with practical experience to make good decisions on intuitive, non-rational and largely incommunicable grounds? There are two things wrong with this conclusion.

First, the claim that, because we need experience and intuitions to make practical decisions, rationality and theory have no role to play, is an inference. The latter claim (that rationality and theory have no use) is supposed to follow from the claim about intuitions and experience. But does it follow? The inference is only a valid one if we make certain assumptions about the relationship between the terms involved: namely, that 'intuitions' and 'experience' on the one hand and 'rationality' and 'theory' on the other are somehow mutually exclusive categories. The use of one in some way rules out the other: if a judgement or decision is 'intuitive' then this means it cannot be rational. If it is based on 'experience' then it cannot be based on 'theory'. Yet these very assumptions are only plausible if certain theories are true – theories about the nature of experience, knowledge, rationality, intuition and the relationships between them. So the conclusion that 'theory is useless' is itself dependent upon the employment of theory and I will argue that the specific theoretical assertions required to generate this conclusion are demonstrably false. The terms 'intuitive thinking' and 'rational thinking' do not represent two different and mutually exclusive types of thought. Properly understood, they are not alternatives at all. Rather, intuition and rationality are both essential components of human thinking and the meaningful employment of each requires the other. The same goes for 'experience' and 'theory'.

It is just not possible to build up a body of experience – especially one which counts as knowledge of a particular context and provides the basis for making decisions within that context – without organising one's experiences in terms of some theory. Understanding, including the understanding necessary to develop sound intuitive responses, requires the organisation of information according to rational principles and that activity requires the construction and employment of theories. To think at all – to infer, to conclude, to recognise, to speculate – requires that we conceptualise our experiences in some way or other: we fit them into some scheme which we spend our lives developing and adjusting and adapting and we do this so naturally, for the most part so effortlessly, that we rarely stop to reflect upon the marvellous complexity of the processes involved. In the same way, the poet and the composer of music rarely pause to consider the complex relationships between symbol and sound that make their respective activities possible. These activities are no less intuitive for being highly structured. To think that they must be is to embrace a false dichotomy. Similarly scientists, mathematicians and philosophers (including logicians) cannot do without sound intuitions. Often one needs to 'sense' the direction in which to look for a proof before one finds it and this is how the most significant advances are made.

Different theories represent different ways in which experience can be organised. They are the conceptual maps which we need to negotiate our world. Just as music is not disorganised sounds, intuitive thought is not disorganised ideas. Indeed, someone with sound intuitions is someone who can make the right links between apparently disparate features of experience and this is an activity which requires in the background a highly developed conceptual map.

This brings us to the second sense in which the conclusion that 'theory is useless' is unwarranted. We all know that a well-trained observer notices more about her environment than someone with an untrained eye. We know that some people are more observant than others. We can ask: what is it that makes a person a good observer? Is there any way I can improve my own observational skills? Just so, it makes sense to ask what it means to be a 'good' decision maker: what type of training is required to develop this particular skill? We do not simply have to 'leave it to individuals with practical experience to make good decisions'. We can ask questions about what sort of individuals we want making decisions and what kinds of processes are likely to produce that sort of person. Each one of us can ask: how do I become that sort of person?

These are not easy questions to answer. They are, in fact, the fundamental questions of ethics and moral education. To live well, to work well, to make the right decisions – these are abilities which may well require practical experience but that is not to say that simply having been alive, or in one's position for a number of years, is sufficient to have developed these abilities: any more than to be a good observer it is sufficient merely to be physically present in a scene and to have one's eyes open.

The value of philosophy

To answer these questions sensibly we need to do philosophy. We need to discuss not simply particular decisions or issues but the processes and assumptions which underlie decision making. At every point in our lives, in all that we think and do, we are influenced by theories, by pictures of our environment and practices, which frame our experiences and shape our attitudes, so forming the necessary background to decision making. For the most part, these pictures remain in the background, treated as too obvious to be worthy of attention, let alone criticism. Yet while some set of background assumptions is necessary, this is not true of any particular set. It is by no means obvious that anyone's basic assumptions are correct: the very fact that people disagree so radically about so many important questions should remind us of this. Indeed, the reason why many debates about matters of morals and politics seem intractable is precisely because the parties involved bring with them different under-lying assumptions, ones which they fail to subject to critical attention and which they often fail to articulate or even to recognise (Loughlin 1998a, pp. 62–6).

To do philosophy is to examine such underlying assumptions: it is to bring them into the foreground, to make them the subject of critical attention. If we are to think competently about the sort of decision makers we want, and want to be, then we must learn how to identify and evaluate such underlying assumptions in the thinking of others but, perhaps most importantly, in our own thinking. We must be prepared to take risks – such as the risk of finding that our most cherished ideas are either foolish or incoherent or in some other way indefensible and the beliefs we base upon them are therefore groundless. This is undoubtedly why there are people who find the very idea of philosophy somehow offensive or disturbing. It is perhaps why Nietzsche saw philosophy as requiring not only intellectual honesty but also 'courage' (Nietzsche 1968, p.114). Nietzsche viewed this form of intellectual courage as a prerequisite for freedom, for the alternative is to allow one's ideas and attitudes, and ultimately one's behaviour, to be shaped by forces which one fails even to perceive, let alone control. It is to waive the right to understand oneself, to decide whether there is anything one would wish to change. To pass up this opportunity is to embrace a fatalistic attitude, rooted either in fear or monstrous complacency. It is like the refusal to approach a mirror. If I am determined never to look myself in the face then I am either afraid of what I might see or else I am rather too sure that I know already.

The process of discovering underlying assumptions is called philosophical analysis.[5] The very fact that certain claims seem plausible, or that certain inferences seem valid to a person, can indicate the existence of a set of background assumptions which may or may not stand up to scrutiny. For instance, we saw how the conclusion that 'theory is useless' when it comes to making decisions was taken to follow from the need for decision makers

to have practical experience and that this implied a commitment to untenable (because unduly simplistic) assumptions
about the relationships between experience, intuition, theory
and rationality. To engage in this type of analysis is to attempt
to discern the hidden commitments in the things people say, the
conclusions they draw, even in the questions they think it
appropriate to ask. Philosophical analysis is often critical in
nature, because it has the goal of liberating thinking from the
(usually unrecognised) influence of false theories. I will say more
about this type of analysis in Chapter 5, but it is worth noting
here that it is a skill, which means it is understood primarily by
demonstration and practice. It is not that skills are 'incommunicable': rather, they are not communicated simply by stating a
set of propositions about them. Like other skills, and the tools
which make it possible to acquire them, analytical thinking
needs to be 'picked up'. It requires training. It is shocking that
many people do not think they need intellectual training. The
fact that the phrase 'thinking skills' sounds faintly absurd to the
modern ear testifies to the shameless intellectual poverty of
contemporary culture.

Any work worthy of the label 'philosophy' should demonstrate the proper techniques of philosophical analysis. In Part
Two, I will analyse the work of contemporary management
theorists, in order to expose and criticise the assumptions of
authors concerning such basic concepts as value, knowledge and
meaning. In the other sections, I will examine the work of
philosophers and bioethicists with similar ends in mind.
Through these exercises I want to begin tracing a map of the
territory typically explored under the headings of 'health services management' and 'healthcare organisation and policy', in
order to determine what, if anything, we may sensibly say about
these topics and how we ought to approach them.

Earlier I spoke of a starting point. I also mentioned the goal of
acquiring a vantage point from which problems could fruitfully
be considered and a method of reasoning with which a range of
problems could be addressed. It is worth saying a little more
about these phrases now, if only to show they were not merely
for decoration. Let us take them in reverse order. The reader
should already have a sense of what is meant by a philosophical
approach to reasoning. She may even have had occasion to wish

that her skills were better developed in this area. Many of us have had this experience: being presented with a set of apparently compelling arguments, we nonetheless feel deeply suspicious; there is something wrong but we can't quite put our fingers on it. This may be because the fault lies not in what is actually said but in the assumptions which underlie what is being said. These assumptions may seem innocent; until now, perhaps, it might never have occurred to us to question them. Yet until we are able to expose them we cannot free ourselves from their influence, so we cannot release our potential to think creatively, to explore alternative conceptualisations of our circumstances, ones which may prove more valuable. We are stuck with the uncomfortable feeling that everything isn't right, but we don't even understand why.

The point in studying philosophical theories (contrary to the impression given by some works of 'applied philosophy') is not to find a set of rules or principles to be mechanically applied, automatically giving rise to good decisions. Rather, it is to acquire a set of conceptual tools with which to analyse problems more effectively, enabling us to find an adequate characterisation of our situation. It is to sharpen up our reasoning skills, equipping us to adapt to new contingencies as they arise. Such philosophical rigour in thought is not meant as a substitute for contextual knowledge and sound intuitions: on the contrary, it is a prerequisite for their development. (This is not to say that only people with formal philosophical training are fit to make decisions. Intellectual fitness, like physical fitness, is something we all possess to some extent: thinking, like running, is a natural human activity. Even so, we need to exercise our powers if we are not to lose them.) This brings us to the idea of a 'vantage point'.

An image from Michael Oakeshott's *Rationalism in Politics* captures the idea of philosophical insight so beautifully that it is well worth repeating here.

> '*It is like the cool touch of the mountain that one feels in the plain even on the hottest summer day.*'
> *(Oakeshott 1962, p. 193)*[6]

I do not mean that the philosophically educated decision maker should be 'miles away' from her immediate situation, that she should have her 'head in the clouds'.[7] The point is rather that she knows the territory: she carries with her a sense of the whole scene, even from her position within it. Her clarity of thought derives from the perspective she brings to practical matters, not from her being at a cognitive distance from the practical. Indeed, she must have extensive empirical knowledge of the context of her decisions if she is to understand what it means to do well in that context.

Traditionally, the type of education required to assume this perspective has been the preserve of the social elite. Nietzsche, who makes it clear that he thinks of his work as being for 'the very few' (1968, p. 114), seems to assume that the vast majority of people are neither capable of, nor do they have any need for, the insight and quality of thought provided by a philosophical education (ibid, pp. 63–4, 92–5). Indeed, he adopts a writing style which seems calculated to keep out the 'riffraff'. Ironically (or, rather, cynically), those who have appealed to populist and democratic rhetoric about the need for 'mass' education, in order to justify some of the recent attacks on traditional academic subjects, take Nietzsche's assumption as read. In demanding that education be 'tailored' to the 'needs of the masses', by being made less academic in order to be properly 'vocational', those who have 'reformed'[8] our education system effectively assume that what the masses 'need' is training in a narrow range of skills appropriate to their station in life. The idea that 'the masses' might receive the sort of good general education which those politicians defending the 'reforms' themselves received is treated as too absurd to be worth considering: if education is to become mass education, then it must at the same time become bad education. What is the point in encouraging people to ask questions not directly relevant to their ability to perform their labour functions? Or as Nietzsche himself puts it, in one of his more obscene moments: 'If one wants slaves, one is a fool if one educates them to be masters.' (ibid, p. 95)

Thus one's view on who philosophy is for is determined to no small extent by one's beliefs about (or, to adopt the now fashionable Blairite parlance, one's 'vision' of) the social order – whether or not one is prepared to own up to those beliefs within earshot of the 'masses' whose 'needs' one presumes to determine. We will return to the relationship between political philosophy and education in Part Four. For the time being, suffice it to say that from my own, rather different, political position, what society needs is more individuals with the capacity to think critically: we need to know not simply what is 'relevant' to perform our functions; we need the ability to *decide for ourselves* which concerns are relevant to us and to do this we need to understand the wider contexts which circumscribe our roles. A society of people who lack this broad understanding, who are only interested in learning what they 'need to know' to draw a salary, is indeed little better than a society of well-trained slaves. We all need the type of general education that was once (and to a large extent still is) the preserve of the elite, if we are to be more than simply items on the labour market.

So what did I mean by speaking of a vantage point? To function as intelligent agents we need to acquire a broad understanding of the forces which shape our thinking. While immersed within a context, we need nonetheless to be able to reflect upon our conceptualisation of that context, to understand why people typically think in the way they do about it. We need to be able to do this without it in any way impairing our ability to react quickly to problems as they arise. Consider the difference between driving through an area you know well and one which you hardly know at all. When you know the area you do not have to stop to think about how to negotiate it: indeed, your knowledge makes it possible to consider the full range of options concerning routes you could take, should unforeseen obstacles present themselves. Just so, as we build up a conceptual map of the territory we want to understand, we cannot simply learn one route through it, if we are really to know our way around. We must understand the broader social and political context within which the health service functions; we must identify and evaluate the ideological assumptions which influence thinking in this area and we must note any discrepancies between ideology and reality – taking note of any limits they place on what we can realistically hope to achieve within our own specific remit. We must learn to think beyond our roles if we are to function as autonomous moral beings within them. Philosophy is for anyone sane enough to want to understand their world.

This brings us finally to the claim about a 'starting point'. No theory can provide a set of decisive conclusions about 'what should be done' in every possible set of circumstances which the reader might encounter. Attempts to apply theory too directly to practice make the same error as the so-called pragmatist who thinks he can do without theory altogether: they oversimplify the theory–practice relationship. The map traced can never be a complete picture. It is up to the reader to fill in the details as she lives her life, using her own unique knowledge of the contexts she encounters. It is important for theory to recognise its limits. It can equip people with crucial reasoning skills and with a broad understanding of the areas it examines. In this sense, it is right that theory should be abstract. But for this very reason, a sound grasp of theory, even when accompanied by the sincere intention to apply it properly, can never be sufficient to live well. We also need specific, contextual awareness.

Theory can only affect the world insofar as it affects the minds and attitudes of human beings searching for just and humane solutions to the problems they encounter. A good theory is distinguished by the way in which it affects people: it should enable them to understand the causes of their problems and to think creatively about them. It should not encourage them to delude themselves with simplistic or bogus solutions. Instead, it should teach them to identify and examine fundamental assumptions critically and with intellectual honesty and to pursue a line of argument to its logical conclusion, however incompatible that may turn out to be with the accepted dogma of the day. So this work not only advocates a certain style of thinking, it also attempts to promote it directly. It advocates an approach to moral education and it also exemplifies that approach. How successful it is will depend, to a large extent, on what the reader proceeds to do with it.

A note on structure

So, the structure of the book is as follows. In what remains of Part One I will look at some of the key theories about the nature of moral thinking and explain my claim that all practical problems are really moral problems. I will begin to sketch a view of the nature of moral reasoning and its proper place in human life but the full picture will not emerge until the final section. (I have my reasons for this – more in a moment.) In Part Two I discuss management theory, bringing out its main ideas and assumptions, tracing its development from its origins as a marketing ploy, popularised by certain business 'gurus', to an all-pervasive and ideologically loaded language, with fluent speakers in all the public services and aspirations to become the adoptive mother-tongue in every region of professional life. This will involve discussing such notions as Total Quality Management, the claim that management is a science and that all organised activities can be evaluated in terms of its key 'principles'. We will see that 'management science' is in fact a pseudo-science, that its proponents are confused about the nature of science and the meaning of evaluative terms and that they disguise their own massive confusions with spectacular flourishes of gobbledegook. The flaws in the approach derive from its attempt to reduce human practices to a set of principles, its attempt to discuss issues that are primarily matters of ethics without doing moral philosophy and its failure even to recognise, let alone to question, the assumptions it makes which are political in nature.

Part Three discusses the nature of applied philosophy and explains the need for a specifically philosophical approach to understanding practical problems, if we are to have a serious and realistic debate about them. This will involve explaining in detail what it means to apply any theory to practice, since there are disturbing confusions about this, even in the writings of some respected applied philosophers. In particular, it is important to reject a popular conception of 'applying' theory in which some completed whole thing, the theory, is somehow 'introduced' into another thing called 'practice' whose nature is treated as theoretically 'neutral' or transparent. As we have seen, all thinking involves the use of some theories, in terms of which our practices are described and evaluated, and the theories we accept help to shape our perception of the reality we hope to understand and affect. The great virtue of philosophical methods is their ability to make our implicit theoretical assumptions the subject of explicit and critical debate. Chapter 5 will incorporate a defence of applied philosophy against those critics who think philosophy has nothing to do with 'the real world', showing their position to be founded upon philosophical assumptions which have been discredited. An important feature of the argument is the rejection of 'irrationalist' positions in moral philosophy, which are seen to embody untenable conceptions of the nature of reasoning and its relationship with intuition and human emotions – conceptions which reflect an erroneous picture of the relationship between theory and practice.

Having explained (in Chapter 5) the nature and importance of applied philosophy, I then examine its limits in the context of the debate about the organisation of health services (Chapter 6). Particular attention is given to that branch of applied philosophy called 'bioethics', which attempts to affect practice in the health services via the direct application of certain principles or ideas derived from philosophical ethics. This might involve the construction of professional codes of practice for certain specified groups, such as clinicians and health service managers, or it might involve the attempt to influence policy makers with philosophical arguments. (The most successful bioethicists sit on government committees offering 'advice' to politicians on how to behave more 'ethically'.) Unfortunately, this attempt to introduce the 'real world' to philosophy also embodies false assumptions about the relationship between theory and practice: assumptions which are founded upon an inadequate characterisation of the context in which decisions about health services organisation take place. These assumptions are shared by health economists, who have contributed significantly to the development of bioethics, with such theoretical devices as the quality-adjusted life year (QALY). The picture of the social world which gives rise to these approaches is so deep-seated, so natural to our pre-reflective consciousness, that it must be viewed as part of the *mythology* of contemporary political culture. The very existence of these approaches threatens to underwrite the conceptions of practice which must change if real advance is to be possible.

By Chapter 7 we should have a good grasp of the depth and complexity of the problem. We need applied philosophy if we are to have an honest and reasoned discussion of the problems of the health service, but the social context in which the service must operate makes the direct application of philosophical principles impossible. Part Four attempts to explain and defend a more subtle and effective way in which rational thought can affect practice. Before we can find the right answers, we have to find the right questions and the key questions we need to ask are: what sort of person can manage well and what are the barriers to decent management and policy? The sort of person to be trusted to practise well is someone with extensive experience of the context of the practice combined with sound intellectual instincts. Thus, the moral problems of practice become problems of education: how do we acquire the right sort of experience and instincts to function well? Chapter 7 outlines a picture of the relationship between moral reasoning and education which is agent-centred (an approach to ethics often associated with Aristotle) and maintains that the goal of education is to produce the right sort of people to face the world. Chapter 8 discusses methods of intellectual training and exercise which can enable individuals to develop and maintain the right attitudes to practice and it indicates ways in which management as a professional group can work to provide the right sort of education to its practitioners. (Education, in this view, is not conceived as something which happens at the beginning of our lives and is then behind us. We should never stop learning and the most important things we learn are not statements of fact but habits of thought and behaviour. This is why it is just as important to maintain the right attitudes as it is to acquire them in the first place.)

However, all honest theorising must be accompanied by a realisation of its own limits. Ethics becomes political philosophy when limits on the intelligibility and effectiveness of moral thinking are discovered to have their roots in a social order which creates barriers to humane and effective practice. Management theory has been implicitly conservative in refusing to discuss the political causes of the problems of the health service. There will be no long-term solution to the broader problems of health service organisation and policy until the social world becomes a more sane and decent place. Individuals and professional groups have a duty to think beyond their official remit, to question the constraints on their practice and to think creatively and courageously about ways in which they can contribute to the struggle for a more decent world.

Such is the conclusion. The astute reader will note as she goes through the text that, while a critical style is adopted fairly consistently throughout – the rationale for this should be clear by now – certain chapters (3, 4, 6) are primarily critical in nature, being concerned with the debunking of alternative approaches to the subject matter. Meanwhile, the positive thesis (the account of moral reasoning, the arguments about education and politics) is developed and defended in Part One, Chapter 5 and Part Four. The reader may wonder why the substantial thesis is scattered across the text in this apparently haphazard fashion. Is the style of presentation purely for effect, like the decision of a 'murder-mystery' novelist to scatter clues about the work, interspersed with red herrings, only to reveal in the final chapter that Jasper is really the killer and all of Henry's suspicious behaviour was due to his tragic and rare personality disorder?

In fact, there are good reasons for organising the argument in the way I have chosen. First, the negative or critical stages of the argument are just as important, just as much part of the substantial thesis, as the positive assertions defended. Indeed, I have serious doubts about the use of the terms 'negative' and 'positive' in contemporary debate: they have ideological over-tones which I bring out and criticise in Chapter 6. To expose a proposed solution to the problems of practice and policy as bogus is to advance an argument. It is to say something signifi-cant and valuable, especially when the solution in question is widely promoted by its exponents, in volumes which make great claims on its behalf and label all who doubt it ignorant or confused. We make a helpful contribution to a debate whenever we ask the right questions, even when those questions serve only to bring out the shortcomings of currently fashionable theories. Such 'negative' arguments are essential for progress. They enlighten the reader, enabling her to avoid errors she might otherwise make and requiring her to think creatively about alternative conceptualisations of the problem. A further, related reason can be explained by returning to the 'novel' analogy of the previous paragraph.

Suppose you learned on the first page that 'Jasper is the killer': what would you have learned? Before you knew anything about

Jasper, before you had followed the development of his character, wondered whether that sort of person could really commit that type of crime, speculated on possible motives, assessed for plausibility the explanations he offers for his behaviour – in general, built up a picture of who he is – the statement that he is the killer would have little significance. It would certainly have no substantial content to distinguish it from the claim that Henry is the killer. If the conclusion is to mean anything, you must understand the materials from which it is formed. Just so, we understand any substantial thesis only if we understand how it develops in the mind of the theorist. A statement of 'positive' recommendations and conclusions, abstracted from the processes of thought and all the considerations which give rise to them, is as useless, as devoid of substance, as a one-line novel which reads: 'There once was a killer and his name was Jasper'.[9]

I have described the approach to ethics adopted in this work as 'agent-centred'. I was drawn to this approach only with some reluctance. Generally, my preference was to debate directly the sort of outcomes we might want to bring about or the sort of principles we should live by, rather than to talk about the sort of people we want around and the sort of people we want to become. It was only as I studied the literature on the management of health services that I came to realise the hopelessness of attempting to approach the topic in my preferred ways. Often I was able to trace the confusions in the work I studied and the superficiality of the solutions offered to apparently reasonable assumptions and goals and it was through questioning these assumptions and abandoning these goals that I came to the approach advocated in the conclusion. Thankfully, we really do live and learn. We cannot really know how good a theory is until we have attempted to use it: application is the test of credibility for any theory, moral theories included.

A theory is defined just as much by what it rejects as what it proposes. A doctrine which excludes nothing asserts nothing. Reading the sections in the order they are presented, I hope that the reader will follow my thinking, experience my frustrations with the literature analysed and search with me for a better alternative. Even if she finally rejects my approach, the journey will have been worthwhile. She can then continue without me.

Chapter 2

The nature of morality

Many writers in the field of 'ethics' (usually the ones who have studied little or no philosophy) think there is an important philosophical distinction to be drawn between the terms 'ethical' and 'moral'. Indeed, the exponents of 'management theory' sometimes chide philosophers for semantic sloppiness on this point, the apparent belief being that the word 'ethical' is a much more technical and academic word than 'moral' (Wall 1994, p. 318). Similarly, student essays often claim that there are telling 'moral and ethical' objections to a particular course of action or policy, suggesting a view that these terms refer to two quite different sorts of objection; or they will condemn a person's behaviour for being not only unethical but, in addition, immoral. Rarely, however, are such assertions accompanied by a clear account of the difference between the terms, such as an illustration of an act that would qualify for one of them but not the other, being at once ethical and immoral or unethical and highly moral.

The reality, of course, is that in common usage the terms are frequently interchangeable. We use them both to evaluate persons and their behaviour: I might express my disapproval of your actions by labelling them unethical, immoral or wrong, but I add very little semantic content to my condemnation by ladling on all three terms at once. That is not to say we can't legitimately construct distinctions between the terms, for instance by stipulating that the word 'ethical' refers to behaviour which conforms to some specified public code – such as the various quasi-legal 'codes of conduct' espoused by professional bodies in medicine, nursing and law. There is nothing philosophically problematic about this, so long as we remain aware that the linguistic distinction, like the code itself, is a human invention.

The problem arises when such codes are used as a substitute for sincere critical thinking about right and wrong, as if the very fact that an 'ethical code' exists can settle a substantial question about how we ought to behave, making one action definitively the right one and another wrong. So, a doctor who disagrees with the official view of the BMA on the subject of euthanasia may have his views dismissed as 'merely' his own, moral position and therefore somehow less significant than the official, 'ethical' position. However detailed and well thought out his arguments may be and however questionable the reasoning behind the official pronunciations, there is an assumption that he should put aside his own views in favour of the dictates of the formal code, even though that may lead him to act in ways he regards as immoral.

Clearly there are practitioners who think that the whole of practical reasoning is a matter of referring to the relevant regulations: if there is a right answer then it will surely be 'written down' somewhere, bypassing the need for independent thought on the part of individuals. This mentality is often portrayed as a responsible recognition of one's own fallibility: 'who am I' to disagree with the official judgements of my ethics committee, professional council or what have you? In fact, there is nothing responsible about it. On the contrary, to think in this way is to abdicate responsibility for one's actions. In life, no-one can 'write down' the answers for you: there is no such thing as a moral rubber-stamp and anyone who claims to possess one displays an arrogance rooted in profound ignorance of the nature of moral existence.

To be a moral subject you must think for yourself. Even if an answer is written down somewhere, the person or persons who wrote it are fallible human subjects also and they have the additional disadvantage of operating at a distance from the specific and immediate problem with which you are confronted. As we have seen (Chapter 1) features of the immediate context might be relevant to determining the right thing to do and, as we will see shortly, even if the authors of a code of practice have extensive factual knowledge of the type of problem which faces you, that is quite a different thing from their possessing moral expertise. At the basis of any ethical code is a set of moral judgements. Since the authors of the code are fallible human beings it will always be an open question as to whether these judgements are correct. If you like, you can use the word 'ethical' to refer specifically to the judgements made by some particular group of people but what you cannot do is escape the responsibility to think for yourself by such linguistic stipulation. 'I was just following the code' is no more a justification for a choice than 'I was only obeying orders'. You would at least need to show that you understood and could defend the moral judgements expressed by the authors of the code, and that they were relevant to the specific situation in which the choice was made. Mindlessness and formalism infect public life at all levels,[10] but they are no substitute for the application of intelligent, critical thinking.

A more helpful distinction between the terms 'ethical' and 'moral' is employed by the philosopher William Frankena. Discussing humanity's sustained efforts to obliterate its own environment, Frankena suggests that the problem may not lie with our 'ethics' but rather with our 'morals' (Goodpaster and Sayer 1979, p. 3). By this he means that it is not the moral principles we espouse or the theories we accept about right and wrong that are responsible for our mistreatment of nature, but rather it is our failure to live by these principles or to act as these theories would suggest we should. Whether or not he is right about this point, the distinction he is employing is clear and in line with the standard uses of the terms in philosophical debate. 'Ethics', as understood by the philosopher, is the systematic study of morality – moral thinking, moral language, moral behaviour. Morality concerns the way we live our lives, the choices we make, the sort of people we are. To ask moral questions is to ask questions about how to live and about what matters in life.

Before making the account a little more precise it is worth considering one difficulty first. There are as many different views about the nature of morality as there are views about how to live and about what is important in life. For a more straightforward subject, like geology, there is at least a broad consensus about the nature of the subject matter, even if theorists differ radically over how to explain its behaviour and the specific methodologies appropriate for its study. In contrast, ethics is one of those subjects so controversial that the attempt to characterise the subject matter is itself a matter of controversy. One problem is that, because there are so many different uses of the term 'moral', it is hard to know which ones to adopt and why. For instance, to some people 'moral' questions concern matters of sexual behaviour and other so-called 'private' affairs, as opposed to 'public' acts performed by individuals functioning in 'official' capacities. So when an American president deliberately orders his bombers to maim and kill, we may 'disagree' with his policy decision but we are not supposed to think of him as an immoral person – even though we easily recognise the unspeakable wickedness of others who commit similar acts of barbarity, often in the name of better causes, but who are not surrounded by the trappings and mystique of public office and the spurious 'authority' it is supposed to generate. However, when the same US president has a sexual liaison with a young intern, leaving no bodies smashed or burned beyond recognition, only then is the man's 'moral calibre' called into question. Only then is he expected to weep on TV and admit to the world that he did something 'morally wrong'.

As with the previous point about the use of the word 'ethical', it is hard to convict people who use the word 'morality' in this way of any philosophical error. As Humpty Dumpty said to Alice, people can use words in any way they like.[11] We can, however, question the utility of restricting the application of the term to any specific subset of human actions. If the actions we perform as part of our 'official' roles have effects on others, why should they be exempt from moral criticism? Again, the point is not so much 'what is the correct use of the term?' as 'what do we want to use the term for in the first place?' If our purpose is to live intelligent and responsible lives, then there is no reason why we should restrict our abilities to evaluate and criticise to some narrow range of choices people might make. What we need instead is a use of 'morality' which does not embody arbitrary distinctions and which is helpful to people in determining the conduct of their lives in any situation they happen to face, including the choices they make while acting within professional roles.

We need to ask: what is morality to mean if there is to be any good reason to discuss it? Put like this, the question suggests its own answer in terms of a defensible working definition of morality as follows. Discussions of morality are discussions about what we have good reason to do and any choice we might make can, in principle, be evaluated in these terms – as either a good choice, one we have reason to make, or a bad choice, one which we should not make. The terms 'right' and 'wrong' only have practical relevance if they are used to denote reasons for choosing or avoiding certain courses of action.[12] To say that an action is morally wrong is to say that you should not do it, which is to say you have a reason not to do it. To say that something matters or has value – be it the natural world or a human life – is to imply, at the very least, that we have good reason not to destroy that thing, which is why it is at least peculiar when politicians who prattle about the value of life order the annihilation of the thing they purport to value.

It would be odd to deny this. Someone who claims to believe that a policy is the wrong one but sees no reason not to continue pursuing that policy is surely confused: it is hard to see what the claim could possibly mean. We use the terms 'right' and 'wrong', 'good' and 'bad' to talk about what we should do, which is to say, what we have reason to do. (Again, what would it mean to say that I should do X but that this gives me no reason to do X?) This is why I stated (in Chapter 1) that all practical problems are really moral problems. For whenever we can ask questions about what we have reason to do, there are various practical options open to us and we can use our critical faculties to think about which options to pursue. Whenever I think rationally about what I should do, I am engaged in moral reasoning. It follows that there is no distinction worth making between theories of rational decision making and moral theories.

Rationality, egoism and postmodernism

Although I have said it would be odd to deny these points, I can think of at least two reasons why people might want to. The first is the influence of a doctrine called 'egoism'. To say that what is right is the same as what I have reason to do is to equate rationality with ethics. This sounds odd to the modern ear because to many people 'rationality' means 'rational self-interest', an idea which suggests that we each have reason to think about ourselves and no reason to care about others, except insofar as their well-being affects our own. Yet morality, surely, may sometimes require us to put the interests of others before ourselves, so ethics, the study of morality, and rationality, the pursuit of self-interest, are surely two different things.

The problem with the line of reasoning just sketched is that it is inconsistent. If egoism were correct then it would follow that we all should be self-interested, in which case it would be false to say that morality requires us to put the interests of others above our own. For what sort of a 'requirement' could this be? Not a rational requirement, if rationality requires me to put myself first. Thus, if egoism is the correct view about rationality, then the only defensible conception of a 'moral requirement' must also be understood in egoistic terms. Morality, as far as the egoist is concerned, is reducible to self-interest: what I ought to do is equated with what is best for me. Self-sacrifice would in that case seem not only irrational but also morally wrong. If you find that conclusion absurd then you need to question the view that rationality means 'the pursuit of self-interest'.

In any case, it strikes me that egoism is a doctrine which has been roundly refuted, many times over.[13] There is no obvious reason why I should be exclusively preoccupied with the experiences and history of one particular object in the world, the one that bears my own name. Indeed, to exist as a subject at all seems to involve taking interest in many things which are independent of and can outlive oneself. I might, with good reason, be concerned for the well-being of my fellow human beings, the welfare of non-human animals, the survival of the natural world and even the continued existence of objects of great beauty.[14] Once the equation of 'rationality' with 'self-interest' has been questioned, it is hard to think of any convincing argument to the effect that it is somehow 'irrational' for me to be concerned about such things, perhaps to the extent that I am prepared to compromise my own material well-being for their sake. If I am not involved in any projects that outlive me, if I never look outside myself, then I am not really living a human life at all. Egoism simply fails to explain all the features of human behaviour that make us interesting. Of course, the egoist can adopt the now familiar tactic of linguistic stipulation. She can insist on calling every action a person chooses to perform 'self-interested', even the choice to sacrifice one's own well-being for the sake of others. However, if any action, even self-sacrifice, is labelled 'self-interested', then it is no longer clear what the label means. As we have seen, one cannot establish any substantial point by playing games with words. (Egoists will often say things like: 'But whatever you do, it must be for some reason', yet it is by no means obvious that the reason in question must be a selfish one. It is just flippant to suggest that because a choice is mine it must have a selfish motive, even when it is the choice to put myself out for someone else.)

Another reason for objecting to the equation of rationality and ethics might be a sympathy with postmodernism. It is difficult to say precisely what 'postmodernism' means since its defenders seem to object to any attempts to pin the term down to any clear set of claims which could then be assessed for their truth-value. Indeed, the term appears to function as a label for a range of doctrines whose only common link is a notoriously impenetrable writing style and a hostility to the ideas of rationality, truth and reality. It does seem fair to say that postmodernists generally are concerned with epistemological questions, that is, questions about the nature and limits of knowledge. For our present purposes, postmodernist thinking is of interest in that it has implications for moral epistemology, the study of what we can know or justifiably assert about what is right and wrong. Such thinking questions the idea that it is possible for individuals to think independently and rationally about any question, including questions about the conduct of their own lives. For the object or purpose of any exercise in rational thought is supposed to be the discovery of some truth – about what is the case or about how we should live. But, it will be objected, the concept of truth has been rendered suspect (or, to adopt the parlance, 'problematised') by the arguments of postmodernists.

I will have occasion to return briefly to the views of such thinkers in Part Four. For the time being, the following general observations will have to suffice. Frequently, in the arguments of postmodernists, perfectly reasonable points about the difficulties in knowing the truth about certain questions, or about the role of language in knowledge acquisition, are followed, quite inexplicably, by bald assertions that it is impossible to know the truth of the matter, from which it is apparently inferred (again with little or no explanation) either that there is no truth to be discovered or that the truth is simply a matter of linguistic stipulation. For instance, Bertens (1995, p. 6) moves from the claim that we need to use language to convey meaning, to the conclusion that we can only ever really talk *about* language:

> '... *postmodernism gives up on language's representational function and follows poststructuralism in the idea that language constitutes, rather than reflects, the world, and that knowledge is always distorted by language* ...'

Bertens offers no clear account of the distinction between postmodernism and the 'poststructuralism' it apparently 'follows', except to point out that the former is 'originally American' and the latter is a product of French 'deconstructionist practices' whose aim is to 'expose' the 'self-reflexivity' of language, meaning 'its failure to represent anything outside itself' (ibid, p. 7). He offers very little explanation, let alone argument, for the astonishing claim that language 'constitutes ... the world', which would seem to imply that everything – trees, birds, soil, clouds, oceans, mountains, solar systems . . . quite literally, anything you care to name – is somehow 'linguistic' in nature and dependent for its existence upon 'the interplay of signification'. So the claim that aeroplanes can fly does not represent a truth about the world, which we can prove conclusively with reference to all the evidence in its favour. For language cannot 'represent' anything other than 'itself' and all experience and knowledge are 'contaminated' by language, so all we can really say is that people who are 'embedded' within a 'scientific discourse' tend to *say* that aeroplanes can fly.

At work here appears to be a rather verbose variant of what is known in philosophy as the 'Berkeleyan fallacy', an error sometimes (rightly or wrongly) attributed to the great 18th-century idealist philosopher George Berkeley in his *The Principles of Human Knowledge*. From the very fact that I can think of a thing it is inferred that the thing must be mental in nature, constituted, as it were, by my own thoughts.[15] This obviously does not follow, any more than the fact that I can walk along the road shows that the road's reality is somehow constituted by my walking along it. The only additional argument 'embedded' within Bertens' new postmodern vocabulary is the claim that there is no such thing as a 'transcendent signifier' (Bertens 1995, p. 6), which means that no term conveys meaning all on its own but rather terms convey meaning by being embedded within linguistic structures. A particular word has meaning by being part of a sentence, which has meaning by virtue of the rules of the language of which it is a part, and the language itself has meaning because it is spoken by a community of human subjects. Yet it is quite possible to agree with all these points without accepting the bizarre conclusion that all truths are truths of language because all reality is linguistic in nature. To say that meaning is a matter of the structural relationships between terms is to make a point about how meaning is conveyed, not about what is said. I can only see things because my eyes are part of the whole physical structure that is my body but it obviously does not follow that I can only really see my own body. Just so, I can only talk about the world because of the complex language system I fortuitously inherit, but it does not follow that the world and all that is in it is therefore a product of my language.

Despite the lack of sound arguments in its favour (indeed, it is hard to see how a view which denies rationality could have any sound arguments supporting it) this type of thinking is the height of fashion in the academic world. Thus in certain academic circles the terms 'reason' and 'truth' are treated as referring to occult entities. No-one admits to knowing what they mean but whatever it is, it must be something altogether distant from ordinary life. Accordingly, the attempt to talk about them is taken as an attempt to assume some sort of supernatural or 'transcendent' perspective, which is promptly declared impossible.

More worryingly, such thinking is beginning to inform popular thought about morality, such that highly controversial and possibly unintelligible claims are being treated as if they were firmly established. As I write, I have in front of me an issue of *The Guardian* which contains a debate between a war correspondent and a theatre critic.[16] The correspondent, Ken Lukowiak, complains about a play in which certain 'real-life soldiers' were invited to give their personal accounts of war. Lukowiak's complaint is that one of the key protagonists, a man called Glasnovic, was a high-ranking official in the fascistic Bosnian Croat Militia, the HVO, a group responsible for some of the most unspeakable atrocities committed during the war in the former Yugoslavia. Lukowiak refers to various eye witness accounts, including his own first-hand experiences while reporting the conflict, as evidence that Glasnovic personally ordered massacres of Bosnian Muslims and argues that his claims, presented in the play, to be an ordinary Croatian soldier are 'a pack of lies'. In the light of this, he questions the wisdom of allowing such a person to present his version of events, unchallenged, to an audience who could not be in a position to know that Glasnovic was, in truth, a war criminal.

What is interesting for our present purposes is the nature of the reply. Defending the play, the theatre critic Lyn Gardener does not dispute any of the evidence in support of Lukowiak's factual claims. Instead, she suggests that these claims are 'irrelevant' because the production company behind the play has always 'embraced the idea' that 'truth is a subjective, lived through, experience', from which it apparently follows that the evidence does not 'invalidate' Glasnovic's testimony, which is 'no less valid' than anyone else's. Indeed, the very fact that Glasnovic has an account to give makes him a 'source' of 'truth', such that the play, simply by presenting a version of what had happened, gave us 'truth in the theatre'. With regard to Lukowiak's moral outrage she comments: 'I do not have Lukowiak's confidence, his certainty about what is right and wrong.' The clear implication is that he is somehow arrogant to feel confident about such things, that his confidence is in fact baseless and unreasonable. If Gardener has any reason to doubt Lukowiak's claims about what actually happened, she gives no hint of this, but several of her comments imply that the distinction between 'truth' and 'fiction' is not clear in her mind.

The very fact that such a response can even be judged intelligible to a non-academic audience, such that it gets into print in a national newspaper, indicates the pervasiveness of the thinking behind it. It is incredible that Gardener can effectively tick someone off for feeling 'confident' that it is wicked to massacre civilians, as if she is somehow taking the moral high-ground by feeling uncertain about this point. At the same time she apparently has absolute confidence in an epistemological doctrine whose meaning is far from clear. Either Glasnovic committed the crimes of which he stands accused or he didn't. (This is an instance of what philosophers call 'the law of the excluded middle', a basic logical principle we abandon only at the expense of our sanity.) If he committed the crimes then by telling a story to the effect that he did not commit them, he is clearly lying and therefore he is not a source of 'truth'. It is by no means certain that 'truth' is a 'subjective experience'. Indeed, it is not clear that this claim means anything at all. Needless to say, Gardener does not explain what it means to 'embrace' this idea: certainly it does not mean to give an honest account, let alone a justification, of the assumptions it embodies.

I say this is worrying because it is a particularly insidious form of attack on moral reasoning, attempting to desensitise our moral capacities by portraying them as a symptom of intellectual naivety. There is nothing reasonable, nothing 'intellectual' about having no moral certainties. Indeed, it is unreasonable not to be certain that some things are morally wrong: for instance, incinerating unarmed civilians because they are not members of your own ethnic group. To say that you lack confidence about such things is to demonstrate not theoretical sophistication but confusion about what matters most in life. Such thinking undermines our most basic moral intuitions with reference to mystifying jargon whose legitimacy is treated as too obvious to defend, such that we are left feeling somehow naive or even bigoted if we try to state the obvious. Postmodernism offers the scientifically unqualified their chance to 'blind people with science'.[17] Do not be blinded. Until the meaning of a claim is made clear and its logical force explained in a way that allows you to assess its plausibility, you simply have no reason to take it seriously. I doubt that the denial of rationality makes any sense and I am not convinced that the exponents of such doctrines really believe nor even know what they are saying. If you find yourself in conversation with such a person, throw a brick at him. My guess is that he will duck, because he knows that he and the brick are part of the same physical reality, whose laws dictate that if he and it should collide at high speed then he will experience physical pain; he also knows very well that physical pain is something which he has good reason to avoid. What is more, he knows all these things without having access to any supernatural perspective. In his heart, he admits that there is nothing mysterious about rationality, for despite himself he possesses it to some degree. Rationality concerns reasons: to construct a rational argument is to find good reasons for a conclusion, decision or course of action. To deny the possibility of rationality is to deny that we can have good reasons to form any conclusion, including the conclusion that rationality is impossible, so any doctrine which denies the possibility of rationality undermines any basis we could have to believe it: it is not so much 'self-reflexive' as self-defeating. Similarly, the claim that there is no such thing as truth establishes nothing except its own falsity.

Facts and values

There is, however, a more credible objection to the very possibility of moral reasoning. I say that this objection is more credible because it does not deny the possibility of reasoning as such: it does not make the self-defeating claim that it is impossible to establish the truth of any statement by rational means. Rather it restricts itself to moral and other evaluative claims, arguing that while it is possible to establish what *is* or *is not* the case, it is not possible to establish any claim about what we *should* or *should not* do. The argument, usually taken to originate in the work of David Hume,[18] goes roughly as follows.

We have a clear idea of what it means for a particular factual claim to be true and we have methods for conclusively establishing that some such claims are true. However, it is not nearly so clear what it means for a value-judgement to be true, nor is it clear how one could go about proving the truth of one's moral position to someone determined to reject it. The point is sometimes put more technically, as the claim that there is a logical gap between statements of fact (which concern what is the case) and judgements of value (concerning what ought to be the case). The latter do not, in any straightforward way, follow from the former. No matter how much knowledge I acquire about the facts in a particular area, this does not make me an expert on the ethics of that area. For moral thinking involves more than simply knowing the facts: it also involves evaluating them and no evaluation of the facts can follow logically from the mere recognition of them. To know what is the case is not to know how to feel about it or how to react to it. That feeling or reaction is something which you have to supply yourself: it is not entailed by any true description of the facts of the matter, however full that description might be.[19]

Certainly, there is something to this. Clearly we do recognise a distinction between facts and values, between our beliefs about what is the case and our beliefs about what should be the case. For instance, you and I might agree that capitalism is the dominant economic system in the world today, yet you may judge that to be an excellent thing while I judge it to be a tragedy. A factory farmer and an animal liberationist might both be in possession of the facts about the ways in which animals live and die in modern farming, yet while the animal liberationist sees the pain and misery experienced by animals as a reason to replace such methods of farming with some less violent way to feed the population, the factory farmer does not. The difference between them is not a matter of either person's being ignorant of some fact. Neither person is in any clear-cut sense 'mistaken' about anything. Rather, it is a matter of what they value. The farmer simply does not treat the suffering of animals as being sufficiently significant to outweigh the difficulties he would undoubtedly experience if he were required to change his practices. The animal liberationist, in contrast, does accord animal suffering a significance capable of outweighing human inconvenience. Is not the difference between them, then, a 'subjective' matter, since it is not settled by the evidence but by their personal reactions to that evidence?

Moral philosophers influenced by this line of reasoning have been led to accept somewhat restrictive definitions of their own subject. For instance, RM Hare (1983, p. v) conceives of 'ethics' as a subject exclusively concerned with the analysis of moral language, the study of what people *say* they have reason to do, rather than the attempt to discover what people really have reason to do.[20] Hare's own work provides a good illustration of the artificiality of this type of restriction, since his analysis of the language of morals, with the help of certain assumptions about human nature, leads him fairly directly to a substantial thesis concerning moral decision making called 'utilitarianism'. (We will return to this theory shortly. For now, suffice it to say that it is not simply a theory about what people say they should do: it provides us with a way of judging the reasonableness or otherwise of what they say and do.)

It is not my concern here to dispute the existence of the 'fact–value gap'. Let us agree that there is a difference between statements of a factual nature (such as 'my mother is unhappy today') and statements with evaluative content (like 'I should do something to cheer her up'). Let us further agree that no statement of the first type logically entails any statement of the second type. What does this mean and what precisely does it prove about the possibility of moral reasoning? To say that the first statement does not 'logically entail' the second is to say that it is possible to assert that the first statement is true and the second statement is false, without thereby being guilty of a *formal contradiction.* I contradict myself if I make claims which cannot be true in virtue of the meanings of the terms involved. For instance, I cannot simultaneously assert that 'Harry is a bachelor' and 'Harry [the same Harry] is married to Sue', since the meaning of 'bachelor' is 'unmarried male'. Thus, the claim that Harry is a bachelor logically entails that Harry is not married to Sue (or anyone else). Of course, no such entailment relation exists between the claim that my mother is unhappy and the claim that I should try to cheer her up. It does not follow that, given enough knowledge of the context in which these claims are made, my belief in the truth of the first statement cannot give me a good reason to believe that the second statement, also, is true.

Consider the statement 'my mother is unhappy today'. I might come to believe this statement true on the basis of certain 'evidence': her facial expressions, the tone of her voice, her mannerisms as she goes about certain mundane tasks. The fact that someone who does not know her so well might encounter the same behaviour but fail to come to the same conclusion shows that the evidence for the claim does not logically entail the conclusion. If that person sees no reason to believe that my mother is unhappy he is not guilty of a formal contradiction but he is wrong, all the same. This point can be generalised to cover any substantial claim about matters of fact. Even the obvious fact that you are now reading a book is not logically entailed by the evidence you have in its favour – the various perceptual experiences (visual and tactile) that lead you to believe it. For there are always alternative possible theories to explain the data of experience. Philosophical sceptics can have great fun constructing such theories, invariably bizarre: for instance, the theory that you are now asleep and having a lucid dream to the effect that you are reading a book about ethics; the view that you have been programmed with a set of false memories and that you are living in a virtual reality machine; even the hypothesis that you are in fact a disembodied brain in a vat. So it does not follow logically from the fact that you are having these experiences that you really are reading a book, since it is logically possible that the 'book' you are apparently reading is just a dream or illusion. (That is to say the claim, however implausible, is not formally inconsistent.) Does this show that you have no grounds to believe that you are now reading a book? Or just that the relationship between evidence and assertion is not one of logical entailment?

Similarly, the fact that the relationship between factual and moral assertions is not one of logical entailment does not show that the facts cannot provide good reasons to accept some moral claims and reject others. The distinction between facts and values is not a matter of judgements about values being 'subjective' in any sense that judgements about the facts are not. In each case, rational subjects are required to make judgements, to 'supply' a conclusion on the basis of the evidence, but this does not imply that any conclusion you care to supply is as good as any other. The fact that 25 witnesses, none of whom has any reason to lie, all say that they saw A stab B; the fact that A had said on many occasions that he intended to kill B; the fact that B's blood was found all over A's knife and on his clothes; the fact that A now says 'all right, I admit it, I killed him': these facts do not logically entail the statement that A stabbed B, but anyone who says they do not give us good reason to think he did is just being silly. (A juror who refused to convict on the basis of such evidence, claiming to have a 'reasonable doubt', would demonstrate not philosophical exactitude but a misunderstanding of the meaning of the word 'reasonable'.) Analogously, the fact that A's action ended B's life prematurely; the fact that it caused B to experience terror and pain; the fact that the only explanation A offers for this action is that B was a 'cocky little nigger': again these facts do not logically entail that A's action was morally wrong or that A is a bad person but they do give us every reason to come to these conclusions.

The fact–value gap, then, is just a species of a more general, logical gap we might call the 'evidence–assertion gap'. As thinking subjects, we are always required to 'go beyond' the evidence available to form conclusions, whether those conclusions are expressed as a judgement about what 'is' the case or as a judgement about what 'ought' to be done. This is so even in relatively uncontroversial cases. We must be able to recognise reasons. In any real situation it is not enough, simply, to learn all the 'facts of the matter' to be a successful thinker. Nor is it enough to know what follows logically from the known facts: logic is an essential component of human reasoning but it is not the whole of human reasoning.

Even in medical education the distinction between 'factual knowledge' and 'reasoning skills' is beginning to be taken seriously, as the profession belatedly acknowledges that the difference between a 'good' and a 'bad' practitioner is not simply or even primarily a matter of who has internalised the most information (Davis 1997). Nor is the formula of 'knowledge plus technical skills plus experience' sufficient to guarantee sound practice since often what is needed is the ability to recognise relevant differences between a given situation and anything one has experienced beforehand (ibid, p. 186).

Rather, what matters is the ability to go beyond the known facts to draw the right conclusions, to infer and also to evaluate, and this involves recognising what counts as a good reason for a conclusion or course of action. The central question, then, is: what does it mean to reason well? How do we distinguish relevant from irrelevant features of a situation in order to determine how we ought to respond? Far from making reasoning impossible, the fact–value gap (or rather, the evidence–assertion gap of which the fact–value gap is a species) brings out its centrality in human life. We are never 'forced' to any conclusion. If we were, the activity we call 'thinking' would be superfluous. In everything we do, in every conclusion we draw, we are engaged in the search for reasons. Reasons are the 'glue' of thinking, binding together evidence and conclusion, without which we would have no means for passing from any experience or thought to any belief or action. Of course, our reasoning may not be sound, in which case we are likely to draw the wrong conclusions on the basis of the evidence. This is why it is so important to think seriously about the nature of reasoning, about what it means to have good reasons for our beliefs and decisions. These are fundamental philosophical questions. (This is why I said in Chapter 1 that we cannot avoid having a position in philosophy, even if it is one we refuse to defend or even recognise.) Traditionally, theories about what counts as a 'good reason' in the realm of 'is' judgements (thinking about the nature of the world) are studied under the heading of 'epistemology', the branch of philosophy concerned with the nature of knowledge, while theories about what counts as a 'good reason' in the realm of human action are studied under the heading of 'ethics'.

This distinction is somewhat artificial, however, since it is not really possible to separate these areas completely. The formation of beliefs is a human activity, which means that any acceptable theory about knowledge and the justification of beliefs must have plausible implications for the conduct of a rational human life. This is one of the reasons why radically sceptical theories (such as the theory that, for all we know, we might really be brains in a vat) could never be taken seriously by any sane person. For there is no defensible conception of 'rationality' which could explain how it could be 'rational' (or even meaningful) to conduct one's life as if one were, or might be, a brain in a vat. A certain amount of 'naivety' about the reality of the objects of experience (that is, the inclination to treat them as being just what they appear to be, in the absence of any reason not to) seems a prerequisite of living a rational life, so we have rational grounds to reject any position in epistemology that is incompatible with such common-sense realism.[21]

Equally, it is not possible to separate ethics from epistemology because any plausible moral theory must incorporate a defensible position in moral epistemology. To 'defend' a theory (in ethics as in any other area) is to show that people can be justified in believing it true, which requires having some conception of what it actually means for theories to be 'justified'. It is not enough simply to present a theory asserting that people should be motivated by factors x, y and z. You must be able to answer the question: but why should anyone believe that theory? As we will see, some initially plausible theories can flounder when it comes to explaining their own epistemological assumptions. (This is probably why certain authors in 'applied ethics' take the 'pragmatic' line and avoid such issues altogether. Why get bogged down with technicalities when you can just make a series of assertions and hope that your readers don't notice you have given them no reason whatsoever to accept those assertions?)

In what follows I will argue that the right approach to moral epistemology makes reference to the distinction between 'knowing that' and 'knowing how' (*see* Part Four) and that without this distinction it is impossible to explain the relevance of moral theory to the conduct of human life. The right moral theory is not the one that proves some set of propositions or general principles in terms of which we then evaluate actions. Rather, it provides us with a method for recognising reasons for action in real contexts and in doing so, it helps us to think for ourselves about how to live. Before reaching this conclusion, however, it is necessary to cross some of the territory often explored under the heading of 'moral theory'.

Reasons, consequences and duties

As we have seen, moral theories are about reasons. They are an attempt to understand what sort of concern is relevant to rational conduct. They ask questions like: is there any characteristic way in which a moral person makes decisions? Can we draw any general conclusions from considering specific cases where we feel fairly clear about what is right – conclusions which could then be applied to more controversial or ambiguous cases? If the reader has any familiarity with the literature in this area she is almost certainly aware of two moral theories:

consequentialism and deontology. These theories (or rather, these types of theory, since these terms are really labels which cover a range of related theories) are worth considering, not simply because they are frequently discussed but because they do represent radically different ways of conceptualising the whole process of moral reasoning.

Consequentialist moral theory explains what we have reason to do in terms of whatever action brings about the best consequences in the situation which faces us. If I want to decide what I should do I must therefore try to find out what is 'best', meaning what has the most beneficial consequences and the least harmful ones. If I am to act responsibly then I must perform some sort of calculation, however rough and ready, weighing up the pros and cons before embarking upon a course of action, and this process of reasoning is characteristic of moral thinking. My actions are justified if, and only if, I have good reasons to believe that they are likely to result in more good than bad consequences. The question then arises as to how one identifies good and bad consequences in the first place.

The most famous variant of consequentialism is utilitarianism. The utilitarian conceptualises benefits (good consequences) and harms (bad consequences) in terms of the effects of actions on the lives of conscious beings. Pain is bad because it is *experienced* as bad. All manner of other mental states (such as despair, anxiety, frustration, depression) are also bad for the same reason. Such bad mental states can therefore, for convenience, be categorised in terms of the general label 'unhappiness'. They are all things that we have reason to avoid because they are intrinsically bad and we know that they are bad on the basis of experience. (This is why utilitarianism is often associated with a position in epistemology called 'empiricism', the theory that all knowledge ultimately derives from experience.) In contrast, some things are intrinsically good: there are many mental states that are inherently satisfying and these can variously be labelled forms of 'happiness'. In moral life, then, we should attempt to achieve a balance of happiness over unhappiness. Hence the much-quoted Millean formula: the greatest happiness for the greatest number (Mill 1983, p. 6).

There is surely more than a grain of truth in all this. Of course, consequences matter when making decisions. No responsible person could fail to consider the consequences of a proposed course of action before embarking upon it and it is eminently reasonable to attempt to ensure that more good comes from one's actions than harm. (What would we think of a person who was not concerned to ensure this; someone who was untroubled by the discovery that his actions had caused more harm than good?) The difficulties in anticipating every possible consequence clearly do not refute this point, although these difficulties are sometimes inexplicably treated as automatically refuting the consequentialist (Donagan 1977, p. 201). What else can the responsible person do but try to foresee the likely consequences of an action, acting on the best information available at the time? In many contexts (certainly in the context of health service organisation) this may well be very difficult but only a predilection for intellectual laziness could lead us to the conclusion that moral thinking should always be easy. Indeed, as the economist Alan Williams points out (Williams 1995, p. 222) it just seems to be sheer common sense that our goal should be to 'do as much good as possible'. His QALY device is designed as an attempt to help policy makers put this into practice in the health service. (As such the thinking behind the QALY is straightforwardly consequentialist, though for some reason Williams seems inclined to fudge this point. For a fuller discussion of the QALY *see* Chapter 6.)

As Williams also points out, it seems equally obvious that the quality and quantity of human experiences should at least be central factors in determining which outcomes should be deemed as 'good' or 'bad'. It is one of the great advantages of utilitarianism that its central principle has application in just about every human situation, from simple interpersonal relationships to complex policy decisions. Whenever I am faced with two or more options, my goal should be to work out which option results in the least misery and the most happiness and to choose that option.

The really problematic feature of consequentialism is its claim that moral thinking is not just primarily concerned with outcomes but that this is all it is concerned with: it is not just that the anticipated consequences of behaviour provide us with good reasons to do some things and to avoid doing others; they provide the only *type* of good reasons possible, such that all reasons are consequential in nature. Opponents of this view will argue that there are other sorts of reason. For instance, we can have duties generated by special bonds or agreements which hold out against the consequences. These duties allegedly generate reasons for action which can override any consideration of a consequentialist nature.

In 1793 the great utilitarian William Godwin outraged his readers by claiming that, if he could only save one person from a burning building and the choice was to save the famous philanthropist and social critic of the time Archbishop Fenelon, or the Archbishop's valet, he would save the Archbishop, even if the valet were his own brother or father (Godwin 1985, pp. 169–70). Godwin's position makes perfect sense from a utilitarian point of view. Obviously it would be terrible for either person to have to die and, of course, if possible Godwin would save both people. Presumably we must envisage a situation in which the two people are trapped and Godwin can only pull one of them to safety before the room fills up with smoke and they all choke, the ceiling collapses or what have you. The likely overall consequences of saving Fenelon are, judged impersonally, much better than those which would follow from saving his valet. For if the valet dies, the effects of this tragedy are likely to extend no further than the valet's immediate circle of family and friends. In contrast, Fenelon's death could have much wider social implications. In a society with nothing resembling today's welfare state (a situation which most contemporary politicians would apparently view as idyllic) the work of great reformers like Fenelon could quite literally make the difference between life and death for many of the poor. Godwin's point is that a person's life is not objectively more important because that person so happens to be related to oneself. 'What magic is there,' he asks, 'in the personal pronoun "my", that should justify us in overturning the decisions of impartial truth?' (ibid, p. 170).

Even so, we cannot help feeling that the life of Godwin's brother or father should be more important *to Godwin* than that of a man he knows only by reputation. As Godwin dragged away the fortunate Fenelon, his father could significantly wonder how *William* could leave him, while Fenelon could not have an analogous thought as a stranger dragged away the valet. Godwin's tirades against 'partiality'[22] betray a shocking (and apparently wilful) ignorance of the importance of the personal and the relational in human life. His conception of 'reason' seems too abstract, too detached from the particular commitments that make us human subjects to provide an intuitively adequate account of moral thinking.[23]

Even leaving aside the relevance of personal relationships, there is another type of consideration to which utilitarian and other consequentialist moral theories seem blind: the fact that there are certain things which no decent person should ever consider doing, under any circumstances. It should not occur to us to do them, even if they were in fact the best thing to do from a consequentialist perspective. Again, an historical example will serve as an illustration.[24] It is commonly held that Lenin's decision to have Tsar Nicolas and his entire family shot following the Russian Revolution of 1917 was an act of mindless barbarity, proof positive of the moral bankruptcy of bolshevism. In fact, this is unlikely. Contrary to the view presented by the popular media, whose presentation of history has all the scholarly rigour of a Barbara Cartland novel, the forces supporting the Tsar in post-revolutionary Russia were anything but romantic heroes. The Russian monarchists were guilty of acts of obscene barbarity, far surpassing anything the communists could achieve in that department, and Lenin was undoubtedly aware that their whole reason for fighting on was to restore the 'legitimate' monarch to power.

It is a central tenet of the monarchist's belief system that legitimacy (the 'right to rule') is passed on through bloodlines. So long as a surviving blood relative of the Tsar lived, the so-called 'white Russians' would have the motive to fight on and the war in all its atrociousness would continue. To end the bloodline, once and for all, would surely strike Lenin as a good way to shorten the war, depriving his main opponents of their key motive to continue, perhaps saving many more lives than were ended by the family's summary execution. In other words, it is at least possible that he had sound consequentialist reasons for his action. Let us suppose (purely for the sake of argument) that he did. While this may make him seem less monstrous, it is unlikely that many of us will find that we now approve of his action. There are some things you just don't do and shooting children as young as three years of age surely counts as one such thing – even when it is likely that by doing so one may prevent others from committing similar atrocities, perhaps on a larger scale. We can't help feeling that, had Lenin been a better person, this 'solution' would simply not have occurred to him. The fact that he could even think of killing the entire family, the children included, shows how brutalised and damaged an individual he had become. We can perhaps understand how war can do that to a person but we still cannot approve of him. We would certainly never wish to *be* that sort of person, to become someone who can think in that way. It somehow comes as no surprise to us that he would then go on to betray the ideals of the revolution by laying the foundations for over 70 years of authoritarian government. That is just what we would expect from someone who thinks it is acceptable to slaughter infants for the greater good.

Notice that this is quite a different sort of problem than the one for Godwin. For this is not contingent upon any special bond. Indeed, Lenin may well have felt a closer bond with the working-class children likely to be the victims of monarchist atrocities than with the children of the Tsar. If we take the intuitions at work here seriously (and it is worth noting in passing that both the arguments against consequentialism so far rely heavily on our intuitive reactions) then the example suggests that it would be wrong to kill a child that one does not know or have any special attachment to, even to save the lives of one's own children. In other words, it identifies a type of consideration quite different from both consequential considerations and personal attachments and one that is potentially in conflict with such considerations when determining action.

The example (or rather, our intuitive reaction to the example) suggests that there are some constraints on action that any rational moral agent will recognise implicitly. Philosophers have labelled these constraints 'deontological' (Nagel 1986, p. 175) since they reflect absolute or unconditional duties we allegedly have to all other human beings; duties which present themselves (to the consciousness of the responsible moral agent) as inviolable rules. These 'rules' are non-consequentialist in nature since they provide us with reasons to act (or, more often, to avoid certain types of action) quite independently of the consideration of the potential consequences of our action or inaction. Such deontological constraints are sometimes claimed to reflect the basic rights of all persons and as such, they place strict limits on the legitimacy of consequentialist thinking. Thus Nozick (1996, pp. 28–33) refers to them as 'side-constraints' upon action. Within these limits we can attempt to bring about the best consequences, so the primary goal of moral inquiry is not to discover 'what is best?' Rather, it is to discover what is *right*, which is determined by what duties we have and how they limit our capacity to bring about good outcomes within the situations which confront us.

There are more variants of deontological moral theory than I can meaningfully discuss here. Most forms owe a great debt to the work of Immanuel Kant (Paton 1972) who claimed that the fundamental principle of morality was the duty to treat persons as 'ends in themselves', rather than as 'means' to an end. Intuitively, what is wrong with killing one person in order to save several other persons is that in doing so you are treating that person as a means to an end, albeit a commendable end. This idea is sometimes expressed by the claim that we should treat other persons not simply as potential recipients of benefits but as individuals worthy of respect. Allegedly the utilitarian fails to 'respect' others by treating them as components of a consequential calculation rather than discrete and unique individuals.

The practical implications of this philosophy are (to say the least) open to interpretation. O'Neill (1986) uses Kantian moral theory to support admirable conclusions about our duties to secure certain basic conditions for all human beings. Kantian and broadly deontological thinking is clearly behind the various incantations of the phrase 'respect for persons' to be found in the writings of authors in the health field, many of whom consider themselves 'anti-establishment' and left of centre. However, in recent history deontological moral theory has very much been a vehicle for the political right, with authors such as Nozick arguing that all forms of welfare spending are immoral. On Nozick's interpretation of Kant, it is wrong to force one person (for instance, through the taxation system) to contribute to the welfare of another (for instance, by getting her to fund the provision of vital life-saving medical services to that other person) since that is to treat her as a 'means' to the other's 'end'. (Remembering it is beside the point that the 'end' in question is commendable.) Followers of Nozick and his style of moralising have therefore condemned all publicly funded health systems for reducing the 'haves' to 'means' for the benefit of the 'have-nots'. For Spicker (1993, p. 35) systems like the British NHS violate the 'stern but minimum demands of morality'.

The main complaint common to this entire family of theories is that, where you have any set of principles or rules that are taken to be strictly inviolable, they seem bound to conflict in some practical contexts. For instance, if you believe that respecting another person requires informing her about the truth with regard to any matter of great importance to her, and you also believe that you should not inflict serious harm on another person, and if both these considerations represent absolute constraints on action, then you simply have no guidance as to what to do whenever you have grounds to believe that the truth will be harmful.

As anyone who works in a clinical context knows, only sheer dogma can sustain the belief that it is somehow impossible that learning the truth can have a serious and harmful effect on a person. The consequentialist can appeal to 'rules of thumb' – general principles which can, for the most part, be expected to have desirable consequences. For instance, it is usually better for people to know the truth since (by and large) we need good information to function effectively in life. However, because the principle of truth telling is, for the consequentialist, just a rule of thumb and not an absolute, he can (and to be consistent, should) abandon it whenever it is likely to produce more harmful consequences than good ones. In contrast, the deontologist cannot consistently appeal to consequentialist considerations to decide which of two supposedly 'absolute' principles she is going to follow when they come into conflict.

A compromise position discussed in much of the literature in applied ethics is a theory called 'rule-utilitarianism'. According to this view we should follow certain general rules whose ultimate justification is that they are conducive to the general good, but in everyday contexts we should appeal to these 'rules' as reasons for action without thinking directly about the consequences. Such rules might include a prohibition against killing and, quite possibly, the invocation to honour thy father and thy mother. Defenders of this view label traditional utilitarians like Godwin 'act-utilitarians'. Act-utilitarianism is defined as the theory that all actions are justified directly by appeal to the general good, rather than by appeal to intermediary principles such as the ones I have mentioned. Turning on their act-utilitarian forefathers, the rule-utilitarians point out that there are obvious advantages to the practice of respecting general rules and in maintaining special relationships with particular persons (such as one's family and friends). Godwin can therefore be criticised *on utilitarian grounds* for failing to recognise the value of such practices.

Whatever plausibility there may be to this criticism of Godwin, the distinction between act- and rule-utilitarianism is probably not sustainable. As Hare (1972, pp. 130–6) points out, in practice the 'rules' in question would have to be constantly interpreted and adapted to suit the specifics of each new situation, to assure that they really were conducive to the general good whenever they were being applied. A person who simplistically followed a rule prescribing truth telling, even when he knew that in doing so he was causing more harm than good, could not consistently appeal to the general good as the justification for his action (Sumner 1981, pp. 98–9). The claim that in all sorts of other contexts truth telling is conducive to the general good would seem to miss the point. It is rather like reasoning that because I live in a part of the world where it frequently rains, such that it is usually conducive to my comfort to wear a raincoat when I go out, I ought to adopt raincoat wearing as a general rule and wear my coat even on the few days of the year when the heat is sweltering and my more flexible compatriots are walking around in swimwear. In other words, the rule-utilitarian seems to ignore relevant differences in favour of irrelevant ones. This is what JJC Smart (Smart and Williams 1973, p. 10) calls 'rule worship'. Remember, the so-called 'act-utilitarian' (in other words, a consistent utilitarian) can adopt rules of thumb and can also attempt to incorporate consideration of the possible long-term effects of a decision or policy. For example, if you are planning to keep the truth from patients in certain circumstances, it is wise not to advertise this with a large plaque on the wall as one of the 'core values' of your institution, since if you let people know in advance that you may mislead them, this will undermine your attempts to do so. It does not follow that you should never mislead people, even when you can do so successfully and when doing so has better (or less harmful) consequences than telling the truth.

Thus the consequentialist might claim that when two allegedly inviolable principles conflict, their real status is exposed. Because they were only ever really rules of thumb, sensible people are not intellectually paralysed when forced to choose between them and they do so in the only defensible way, by weighing the consequences of the alternative options open. He might add that the intuitive objections raised above were drawn from highly unusual situations and have little or no application to the realm of policy decisions. However important special relationships may be in everyday life, a health services manager who used his influence to get preferential treatment for his mother, or for someone to whom he owed a favour, would not be viewed as a model son or as a shining example of personal integrity but as a corrupt manager. Similarly, in the context of policy making, people may have to consider options that would normally be viewed as unacceptable. While it may normally be impermissible to act in a way that leads to another person's death, a resource allocation decision involving medical services might in principle lead to the death of some, even if it ensures that others may live. Might it not be that consequentialism is the right theory in the context of policy making?

This is an appealing argument, but there are various responses open to the deontologist. She may point out that any intuitive plausibility a theory has in a specific context (such as public policy formation) does not necessarily prove it is the right theory. In general it is recognised that false theories can sometimes appear to give good explanations of specific cases, but the real test of any theory is how it fares over a wide range of cases. Aristotle's physics 'explains' why solid objects have a tendency to fall to Earth, but because the theory fails to explain so many other physical phenomena we do not conclude that it is 'right in the context of falling objects', but that it is the wrong theory. So we conclude that its explanation of the phenomenon of objects falling, though initially appealing, is not in fact the right one. While we have seen there are significant differences between (on the one hand) scientific thinking and other forms of reasoning concerned primarily with discovering facts and (on the other hand) moral thinking, we have also seen that the difference is not a matter of one being 'rational' in any sense that the other is not. In each case subjects have to make judgements on the basis of evidence. Since weak standards of evidence and reasoning are not acceptable in science, it is not clear why they should be acceptable in ethics either. So you cannot just dismiss the general objections to the plausibility of consequentialist moral theory by pointing out that in some contexts (ones which perhaps conveniently involve your own practice) it can sometimes throw up plausible implications. Specifically, if you are a manager and you choose to be guided by a theory which (a) you could not apply in any other area of your life and (b) you could not expect other professionals with whom you deal (such as medical doctors and nursing staff) conscientiously to accept, then you cannot plausibly claim that you have the right theory and hence you cannot appeal to that theory as a justification for your decisions.

In any case, it is by no means obvious that consequentialism has consistently plausible implications, even in the context of health services organisation. How many people would vote for a policy of killing certain healthy citizens to harvest their organs, if that policy were found to be the most efficient way to organise the health service in that it saved more lives than it cost? John Harris has actually advocated such a policy in his notorious essay *The Survival Lottery* (Singer 1990, pp. 87–95). Harris argues the case independently of any commitment to consequentialism, but a consequentialist would surely be committed to supporting Harris's position, while most of his readers treat this implication as sufficiently absurd to cast doubt on the credibility of the theory.

The role of intuitions

What have we established, then? Simply that there are radically different types of concern at work in moral thinking. There are various kinds of reason for action and the consequentialist seems to be wrong in thinking that all reasons to do or to avoid doing something boil down to one category of consideration, the likely consequences of a proposed course of action. That is not to say that such considerations will not often (perhaps even most of the time) rightly be foremost in the mind of the rational decision maker. It is just to say that there are other categories of reason, including reasons generated by special relationships and perhaps even non-consequentialist duties of a more general nature, such as those expressed by the deontologist's 'absolute principles'.

Note that it is not obvious that such concerns have no place in professional life. Loyalty to one's colleagues, clients and even one's employer can sometimes figure heavily in the moral thinking of responsible people. When a person has to choose between preserving the integrity of such professional relationships and doing what is likely to produce the best consequences overall, the choice can present itself as a serious dilemma. Also, the deontologist is probably right to point out that there are some possibilities which simply should not occur to us: such as solving the problem of a shortage of organs for transplantation by lobbying the government to kill certain individuals (perhaps criminals or the economically unproductive) in order to harvest their organs. The idea just strikes any decent person as too absurd to contemplate and, far from being an irrational prejudice, it is probably a precondition of rational life that there are some limits to what we view as 'thinkable'. For we would rightly view with some degree of suspicion any person who saw this possibility as a 'viable' option worth exploring.[25]

The trouble is, we still have no basis to decide between these different types of concern in cases where they conflict. I will eventually argue that it is a mistake to expect to develop a theory which will decisively resolve all such conflicts. Rather, the goal of studying moral theory is to enable us to find the right answers for ourselves. We undertake the intellectual exercise for the same reasons that one might undertake physical exercise – primarily for the effect it has upon ourselves, in producing a certain fitness for the tasks which face us.

I say I will 'eventually' argue these points since I do not expect this conclusion to seem even vaguely satisfying at this stage. For the moment I want to employ a tactic so common in philosophical argument that it must be seen as a definitive feature of this whole style of thinking. I want to step back from the debate so far and reflect upon the form which it has taken. It is worth noting that in assessing the credibility of the moral theories under discussion, it has been necessary to examine the implications of the theories for their intuitive plausibility. A theory which yields profoundly counter-intuitive implications is for that very reason called into question. How else could we assess such theories? A person with no moral intuitions at all would be a person with no capacity for moral reasoning, since he would have nothing which he could recognise as a starting point for his thinking. For him there could be no moral data. Imagine someone who could see nothing intuitively wrong with inflicting intense pain upon a helpless victim. How could such a person be capable of understanding, let alone evaluating, the thinking behind utilitarianism?

Yet for this reason it can be argued that the debate has a serious methodological flaw. To recognise a good theory, and to be able to apply the correct methods for identifying problems for specific theories, it is necessary to have developed sound moral intuitions. However, if we already have sound moral intuitions then what do we need moral theories for, and if we don't already have sound intuitions then how can studying such theories help us to acquire them? Either we can't know which is the right theory (if we lack sound intuitions) or we don't need to know (since we already have sound intuitions to guide our actions). In other words, the theories we have considered so far flounder on methodological (specifically, epistemological) grounds. To think well about moral questions it seems to be both necessary, and sufficient, to have developed sound moral intuitions. We need, then, to give more critical attention to the faculty of intuition. Theorists who have put intuition first in the study of moral thinking include Moore (1903), Pritchard (1949) and Ross (1939).[26]

Moore is famous in philosophical circles as a critic of the utilitarian JS Mill, whom he condemns (along with several other well-known philosophers) for committing something Moore (1903, p. 10) calls the 'naturalistic fallacy'. According to Moore, this fallacy involves treating moral terms as referring to natural properties, like pleasure and pain. Moore reasoned that moral terms like 'good' cannot refer to any natural property, since it is always logically possible to ask the question of any natural property 'is it good?' This is sometimes referred to as the 'open question argument', which Moore triumphantly declared to be as thorough a refutation of any theory as one could ever hope to find (ibid, p. 66).

It is really not clear to me why Moore saw this point as so destructive to the work of Mill. For while it is logically possible to claim that such things as misery, agony and despair are 'intrinsically good' (that is to say, one can do so without being guilty of a formal contradiction) it is surely not reasonable to say this. Analogously, it is an 'open question' as to whether the table in front of me really exists since (as we have seen) it is logically possible to deny this. But anyone who seriously thinks that the table might not be real, or that agony might not be a bad thing, requires the services of a psychiatrist, not a logician. Mill's substantial moral thesis does not require the claim that 'bad' means 'pain', simply that the fact that something is painful always gives us a reason to view it as a bad thing (in the absence of any greater good which might outweigh the badness of the pain). Indeed, Moore's own substantial moral position is very similar to Mill's in this respect. He views certain experiences – such as 'the pleasures of human intercourse and the enjoyment of objects of beauty' (ibid, p. 188) – as intrinsically good and argues that we ought to do whatever 'will cause more good to exist in the Universe than any possible alternative' (ibid, p. 147). Moore's differences with Mill concern matters of logic and epistemology: questions about the meaning of moral claims and how we know them to be true. He reasons that, if moral claims are not claims about natural properties then they must be claims about 'non-natural properties'. The word 'good' just refers to the (non-natural) property of goodness and we know that a specific situation or state of affairs displays this property by intuition.

While I do not think Moore's position is nearly so silly as some contemporary philosophers make it out to be, there is clearly something wrong with his argument. It is unhelpful to translate the claim that we have good reason to avoid such things as pain into a claim about 'non-natural properties'. Suppose we agree that I know by intuition that 'the pleasures of human intercourse' have the non-natural property of 'good-ness'. A wilfully ignorant person could still ask why he has any reason to desire things which have that property. The answer, of course, is because it is just obvious. But we could have given that answer in the first place, without appealing to the bizarre idea of a non-natural property. If you do not see that you have good reason to desire such things as harmonious relations with your fellows and to want to avoid such things as pain and anguish, then you are not functioning as a rational moral subject. In some way you are going wrong. Similarly, if I have all the right perceptual experiences but fail to come to the conclusion that the table in front of me is real, then in some obvious way I am going wrong.[27] To explain this we do not need to posit that when I perceive the table I also perceive a non-natural property of 'reality', which somehow attaches itself to the table. Instead, we need a defensible theory of rationality to explain how I come to recognise such things.

Just as Moore accuses Mill of the 'naturalistic fallacy', so he stands accused of something called the 'referential fallacy', the view that all meaningful terms must refer to some thing or property. For he concludes from the fact that 'good' does not refer to a natural property that it refers to some other kind of property, which he can only think of as 'non-natural'. This does not follow because there are many meaningful words that do not refer to anything. For instance, the terms 'and' and 'the' do not refer to anything, but they are meaningful because they play a role in the construction of meaningful sentences. Similarly, the word 'good' might not refer to anything, but rather we might use it to express our approval of specific situations or actions. (We will see in Chapter 4 that contemporary management theorists commit this fallacy when they construct theories about 'quality'.) What matters for the purposes of moral reasoning is whether or not we have any good reasons to approve of one thing rather than another. To think about this we need to consider substantial questions about what sort of people we should be. It strikes me that Moore could not approach this question in the right way because he was too preoccupied with linguistic analysis. It is absolutely right that philosophers should be concerned with language and meaning, but philosophy for much of the 20th century displayed an obsession with these areas, to the exclusion of all others.

The group of theorists who first identified the referential fallacy shared this obsession with language. These theorists were the emotivists, whose arguments we will have occasion to look at in Chapters 3 and 5. It is worth noting that there are other similarities between Moore and his critics. The emotivists treated moral language as functioning purely to express non-rational reactions. As such, moral claims were treated as unsusceptible to rational debate, leaving little scope for meaningful moral argument. Since the intuitionist position, as characterised so far, states that we 'just know' that certain things are right, it effectively leaves as little scope for theoretical argument about what is right and wrong as the emotivist view. The only difference is that the intuitionist seems to make the additional claim that his reactions are the right ones. He cannot meaningfully defend this claim since unless you already share his intuitions you could not be capable of understanding his defence.

This is clearly unsatisfactory and, as I have indicated, one of the reasons why is the preoccupation with language. Moore was concerned to show how we could know that certain moral propositions were true, such as the claim that certain types of thing are 'good'. He was attempting to give an analysis of the meaning and truth-conditions of sentences which contained moral expressions. This led him to search for moral knowledge of a propositional nature: knowledge that certain propositions are true. I will argue (Part Four) that moral knowledge is essentially practical in nature, and that the goal of moral thinking is the acquisition of a certain sort of skill: a form of 'knowing how' rather than 'knowing that'. Only if we think in this way can we give a meaningful account of the role of both intuition and theories in moral thinking. We cannot construct a mechanism to obviate the requirement for individual subjects to think critically about each new situation they face, but we can develop our capacities to make good, informed judgements, where being 'informed' involves much more than passively internalising certain facts. It involves developing an adequate conceptualisation of the nature and scope of the problems which face us and to do this we need a certain sort of intellectual training.[28]

This training should help to develop our thinking skills, enabling us to identify and analyse the different types of concern that present themselves in any given context; to discover the relevant similarities and differences between this situation and others we are aware of; and also to recognise those situations in which there is no adequate resolution such that any decision must be arbitrary – often because the circumstances in which we are forced to practise make it unreasonable to expect us to find an adequate resolution. That is not to say we should be practically paralysed, but that we must learn how to face such situations with honesty, rather than treating the admission that they exist as a sign of personal failure on our own part. We must learn to take responsibility for that which we control, but also to locate responsibility in the right place where there are features of a situation which we do not and cannot control. This is what is known as realism, an attitude persistently and shamefully discouraged in the jargon-ridden, positive-focused world of contemporary management theory. It is to that world, sadly, that we now must turn.

Part Two

The morass of
management theory[1]

Chapter 3

The illusion of quality[2]

Some years ago I became interested in certain peculiar developments in the world of health management. I became aware of a body of literature whose goal appeared to be the creation of a new and rather strange language to describe and evaluate practice. I soon learned of the existence of courses designed to teach health service workers to use this language, which originated in the world of business and which, according to its defenders, was capable of application to every organised human activity.

This language was associated with an approach to practice which its exponents described variously as a 'movement', a 'management philosophy', a 'leadership paradigm' and a 'cultural transformation' (Al-Assaf and Schmele 1993, p. ix) as well as a 'science' (ibid, p. 209) with its own unique 'principles' and 'methods' and an 'educational experience that infiltrates throughout (*sic*) the organisation and involves everyone – staff and management' (ibid, p. 29). A key claim of this new 'science' is that there are 'basic organisational criteria' in terms of which literally every complex organisation (whatever its goals) can be successfully analysed and evaluated (Berwick 1993, IHSM 1993, Laffel and Blumenthal 1993, Peters 1992). Another key claim is that the concept of 'quality' is fundamental to evaluation, such that we can learn what it means to do well in any area by learning what quality is and how to make it part of the 'process' and 'outcomes' of our activities (Al-Assaf and Schmele 1993, p. v). (As we will see, these two claims are closely related.) Thus management theorists who apply their 'philosophy' (or 'science' or 'paradigm' or 'culture') to health describe quality as a 'cornerstone' of healthcare (Al-Assaf and Schmele 1993, Brooks 1992, Peters 1992)[3] and this 'discovery' is heralded as a conceptual revolution (Hill *et al.* 1990, Joss and Kogan 1995, PA Consulting

Group 1989). As two skilled users of the new language note (Joss and Kogan 1995, p. 5), 'quality' has changed its connotations since the early years of the 20th century, when it was a term associated with 'exclusivity', to become a much more 'democratic' word. Where once 'quality' was a rare thing, it is now found all over the place and the word appears in much of the contemporary literature on evaluation almost as frequently as the definite article. So there are 'quality circles', 'quality continua', 'quality shadow structures', 'quality loops' and 'quality spirals' (Miles *et al.*, 1995). Another characteristic of the new language seems to be a fondness for emphatic words such as 'total': so we have 'total quality', 'total cost management', 'total service delivery concepts' and 'total commitment' (to total quality) (Al-Assaf and Schmele 1993, Joss and Kogan 1995).

Expertise in, and absolute dedication to, Total Quality are often stated as prerequisites for posts advertised in health services management and the subject 'Total Quality Management' (TQM) is offered by management courses at many universities. Nurses can gain qualifications in the discipline of Quality Assurance and health authorities employ people to 'develop', 'facilitate' and 'co-ordinate' quality within their organisations. Resources are invested in workshops, training days and management committees, as well as in articles designed to proclaim the worth of these assorted gatherings of human beings who share a 'commitment to quality'. Large sums of money are spent on the discussion of how to achieve this thing called 'quality' or (more often) of how well it is already being achieved and of how much better still things are yet to become.

There are 'quality engineers', the 'experts' in the new subject called 'quality science' (Berwick 1993). Because 'organisational quality' is 'a managed process' (Brooks 1992, p. 18), 'quality science' is treated as a species of 'management science' and the theorists of this new science call for the use of 'industrial quality management science' (IQMS) in all 'service industries', including the health service (Laffel and Blumenthal 1993).

It soon became clear to me that the approach to practice which this language embodied was palpable nonsense. As I waded through the texts and journal articles it struck me that its exponents understood neither science nor evaluation and that they were employing language not to clarify or 'enlighten', as they claimed, but to mystify and mislead. I also noticed that they were meeting with some resistance from bewildered or cynical practitioners (Darbyshire 1993, Miles *et al.* 1995) and that there were ideological underpinnings to the struggle.

Unfortunately, as a philosopher, I was not supposed to be interested in this sort of thing. On the one hand, the ideologues of the new approach to practice would undoubtedly say (as they since have) that a philosopher cannot possibly have anything 'relevant' to say to 'practical' people like themselves. On the other hand, many philosophers sneer at such social phenomena, which seem to them to be rather too empirical to raise any interesting conceptual questions. The phrase 'shouldn't you be doing sociology?' is used by such philosophers to disparage colleagues who study areas they consider unworthy of philosophical attention. Apart from indicating outrageous contempt for a serious academic discipline, this betrays an attitude in keeping with that of the so-called management theorists, that philosophy should have nothing to say about important questions which affect real life. Do they think it is impossible to think clearly and analytically about such matters or that evaluative questions cannot be answered rationally (making it impossible to give a rational response to any question about how to do anything well)? As we will see (Chapter 5) some of them do think all of these things or at least, they subscribe to doctrines which seem to imply them.

Since I began to write on such matters, the new 'management thinking' I found increasingly disturbing has continued to colonise human society, taking hold of public institutions and even the rhetoric of public debate.[4] It has certainly gained a lot of ground in the world of education. It is my hope that, as these philosophers collate the responses to their 'student evaluation feedback questionnaires', write out their lists of 'learning outcome targets' and sit in seemingly endless meetings with their academic colleagues, trying to implement the latest nonsensical dictates of a management increasingly indifferent to academic matters but immersed in the new rhetoric of 'quality' they pause to reflect on the old adage about the holocaust[5] . . . then they came for me. So long as other sectors were forced to talk nonsense about evaluation, philosophers did not consider it their job to point out the philosophical errors underlying the nonsense. When the nonsense came to the new universities, it still did not matter to those working in the old. Now it is finally colonising every aspect of professional life. They are coming for you, professor.

In what follows I attempt to spell out the essential features of this so-called 'management theory', using articles published over the last 10 years (at the time of writing) to illustrate its key assumptions and inferences. The documents are therefore selected for attention on the basis of their practical orientation (they either make recommendations or actually describe attempts by the authors to put management theory into practice) and the fact that they are fairly representative instances of the genre. This is in no sense intended to be a 'comprehensive review'. If the reader is a management theorist, 'industrial quality scientist' or 'quality engineer' who feels I have missed out her favourite article or text then I will apologise – but only after she has apologised to me and to thousands of other public sector workers for the damage which she and her kind have done to our working lives. I will argue that the whole approach is conceptually flawed and that its exponents cannot give a coherent account, even of their most fundamental ideas.

Of course there are important questions to be asked about the organisation of public services and of course workers in these areas need to develop a language in which to debate these questions. (More accurately, they need to develop their own languages in which to evaluate these practices, since there is no reason to assume, as management theorists do, that concepts imported from one practice will be suitable to evaluate any other.) In Part Four I will say something about the sort of debate we should be having about such matters.

It is possible to talk and to think sensibly about management; it is just that most management theorists fail to do so and the last thing you need if you are to 'manage well' is to learn what is called 'management theory'. The health service and the public services in general need critical thinkers, able to reflect on the problems of their own practice with acuity and intellectual honesty, not decision makers whose specialist areas are in jargon and the creation of paperwork. If only one person reads the arguments of this section and feels better armed to criticise the nonsense, then the work will have been worthwhile. If enough of us feel that the rot must stop, then there is still a chance that it will.

Hollow foundations

Let us begin by examining the intellectual foundations for this new discipline of 'quality management'. What exactly do the new enthusiasts for 'quality' mean by this word? What is this property that they claim should be pursued, managed, directed and above all demonstrated throughout the health service? Remarkably, while there is widespread agreement that 'quality matters', that its presence in the health service is extremely important and even that its absence costs substantial sums of money,[6] there is little agreement over what this thing is that matters so much, nor, in all the 'quality' literature, are there any attempted definitions of the concept central to the discussion that could stand up to serious scrutiny.

Instead, the debate about how to achieve quality is phrased in a pseudo-intellectual 'management-speak', whose quasi-economic ugliness fails to disguise a shocking lack of precision. This language is permeated by platitudinous declarations of deeply held beliefs in, and an absolute dedication to, 'total quality'. It seems that when one's explanation of a concept is equivocal, unequivocal commitment to it will do as a substitute, so writers testify to their conversion to quality in much the same way that the converts of American evangelists publicly and stridently affirm their faith.

As we have seen, along with the increase in talk about 'quality' comes an interest in such apparently related concepts as that of Total Quality Management, Continuous Quality Improvement[7] and the Quality Management Maturity Grid – a device designed to 'diagnose' the level or extent of quality within an organisation by examining 'the continuum of quality awareness' (Crosby 1979, pp. 32–3, Jones and Macilwaine 1991, p. 21). Unlike such better known continua as the space–time continuum, through which physical objects move, the continuum of quality awareness exists within institutions, or at least within those described as 'service agencies', and the consciousness of these agencies moves through it. Suitably qualified managers can intuit the position of their service agency with respect to the continuum, placing the institution at one of five stages of quality development.

In an article entitled 'Diagnosing the organisation: one health authority's experience of Total Quality Management', published in *The International Journal of Health Care Quality Assurance* (Jones and Macilwaine, 1991), two senior managers in the Waltham Forest Health Authority chart the movement of their authority through the continuum from Stage 2 (they had presumably already passed Stage 1, 'Uncertainty', before the period their article describes) through Stage 3 and towards the dizzy heights of Stages 4 and 5 ('Wisdom' and 'Certainty'). After the obligatory assertions that the commitment 'from the top' to Total Quality Management 'was total', they characterise Stages 2 and 3 in the following terms:

> '*Stage 2: Awakening. A quality assurance team is established. Management becomes committed to quality.*
>
> *Stage 3: Enlightenment. Corrective action and communications are established. Management becomes committed to quality.*' (ibid, p. 21)

Since management had already become committed to quality by Stage 2 it is not entirely clear how it can also 'become' committed at Stage 3, but this is a minor point. What is interesting is what in fact was done by the newly established 'quality assurance team' to 'enlighten' the organisation. According to the authors, a letter was sent out to 300 people, all of whom were either managers, consultants, senior nurses or 'professionals allied to medicine', asking them to say what they thought should be done to 'improve quality'. The authors admit that the response to this letter was poor, but explain that there was an epidemic of the 'flu going around at the time (ibid, p. 22).

Out of the total of 51 replies received, the quality assurance team were able to compile six tables of 'quality issues' and to develop a 'District-wide Quality Agenda' (ibid, p. 24). The quality issues identified included such things as improvement in decor and signposting and the material benefits of the exercise, in terms of money set aside to deal with perceived problems, were, the authors concede, 'fairly small'. (For some reason they do not say exactly how small, but instead tell us that this sum of money was 'designated as the facilitation fund'.) In other words, having made certain minor changes, in response to some 51 replies to their initial letter, the Waltham Forest Health Authority felt able to claim that it had 'clearly demonstrated' a 'commitment to excellence'. Nowhere in the article do its authors explain what conception of quality justifies their claim that this exercise in collating 51 responses to a letter constitutes demonstrating quality or showing that one is enlightened about quality. All they tell us about quality is that it should be 'management led' and 'demonstrated' and that an important reason for having it is that it enables an authority to 'build on its . . . good reputation'. (Which seems to suggest, significantly, that there is not so much point in having quality unless you are also *perceived* to have quality.)

However, the exercise is proclaimed by the authors as 'worthwhile' and 'valuable' because 'it pushed the organisation into the third stage of enlightenment' and because it was followed up by the creation of 'an ideas bank for internal customer surveys' and a 'quality news sheet' which became part of the staff newsletter. The article begins:

> 'Born out of the deeply held conviction of the District General Manager (DGM) that quality matters, the Total Quality Management (TQM) approach to quality was adopted in June 1989 by the Waltham Forest Health Authority.'[8] (ibid, p. 21)

They do not explain why the belief that quality matters should 'give birth' to the view that quality should be analysed as a function of management, but their inference is entirely typical. There is general agreement amongst writers on this subject that the development of quality, though 'everyone's business', is primarily the role of senior management, hence:

> *'Total Quality Management requires that there be a management-led commitment to excellence which must be clearly demonstrated.'*

This comment echoes the insistence by two more health service managers, writing in the same journal (Kelly and Swift 1991, p. 26), that in their organisation 'Quality was being led from the top'. Quality is something that has to be 'managed', hence the swift move by Jones and Macilwaine from the demand that quality be 'assured' to 'the Total Quality Management (TQM) approach'. Or as another defender of TQM, Tessa Brooks (1992, p. 18), puts it:

> *'While quality has always been a cornerstone of health provision and an essential, if implicit, component of professional training, it is only in the last few years that real interest has been expressed in the idea of organisational quality as a managed process. With the post-Griffiths development of general management and total service delivery concepts, an environment is being established in which TQM thinking becomes both attractive and relevant.'*

Leaving aside for the moment the ritualistic nature of the 'cornerstone' comment (in what sense, precisely, has quality been both essentially and implicitly a 'cornerstone' for so long?), this statement invites the question, to whom is 'TQM thinking' attractive/relevant, and why? The answer to the first question seems to be: to those involved in administration. The answer to the second question might be because, however many surveys are undertaken, in practice it is senior administrators who decide what does and does not count as quality, an exercise they call 'standard setting' (Kelly and Swift 1991 p. 27). No surprise, then, that they are unclear about the criteria for standard setting: why limit oneself when setting standards by explaining in overly precise terminology what it is that one is trying to achieve by setting them? If people knew what quality was, then they might end up refusing to accept that the products of one's 'initiatives' were indeed quality products.

The mentality at work here becomes clearer still when we recall the historical origins of this 'quality' jargon (to give it the sort of name it might give itself, let us call it 'Qualispeak'). As the authors of a report on 'The quality initiative in the NHS' explain, quality was 'rediscovered' in the 'new political context of the 1980s' by certain 'gurus' from the world of commerce (Hill *et al.*, 1990). These gurus came up with what, for them at least, has been the very profitable idea of 'orientating' business to the idea of quality or 'quality culture' and with governments in the UK and the US determined to subject every aspect of human life to the 'discipline of the market', it was only a matter of time before the latest fad in the world of business became a new ideal for the health service.

What was it that these writers rediscovered, which presumably had until then been lost? An adequate definition of quality? As Brooks (1992, p. 18) admits, in another piece of fluent Qualispeak:

> *'More recent academic writings on the subject . . . accept a complexity of experience in pursuing quality management and . . . [they] accept the discontinuities and discomforts that attend progressive cycles of real advance. It is clear that a simple set of principles and processes cannot be applied across organisations facing radically different external and internal circumstances.'*

Stripped of jargon, this appears to say that there is no definition of quality, nor any formula for how to achieve it, that can be applied even to different types of commercial enterprise, let alone transferred from the context of business to that of healthcare. This would surely make the idea of systematically introducing 'quality management' into the NHS strictly impossible, since one cannot *systematically* introduce an indefinable and apparently ineffable property into anything. Nonetheless, and as if it follows directly from the above comment, Brooks goes on to praise the ability of business analysts 'to define quality as a recognisably delivered entity in the perception of clients or customers'.

Again, it appears that the only substance to the concept of quality is to be found in the fact that some people (here identified as 'clients or customers') perceive a product or service as having quality. Thus Kelly and Swift (1991, p. 26) also stress the need for quality to be 'recognised as an integral part of each department's operations' and the importance of services appearing 'attractive' to 'customers/patients'. This no more provides an adequate definition of quality than the purported definition in 'The quality initiative' report:

> *'Quality is taken to refer to one or more attributes or characteristics of a service which are important enough to be identified and specified.' (Hill et al. 1990, p. 19)*

To define a word is not to say what it refers to: the term 'man' might be said to refer to anything which is a man, but this is not a definition of the term.[9] To define it we must say what the term means. A good definition would help explain what the term meant to someone who did not already know and would serve as a guide to future usage, ruling out some uses in advance by distinguishing appropriate uses from inappropriate ones. If the writers are saying 'quality' means 'certain attributes' then they are simply confusing two senses of 'quality': if a thing's qualities are simply its attributes then they can include 'being awful', but the writers are looking for a sense of quality given which to describe something as having quality or qualities is to praise it. So if the definition is not to be sheer nonsense then it must put all the weight on the word 'important', in which case it is totally vacuous: for how do we decide which attributes are 'important enough to be identified'? If we can decide what is important without appealing to quality then the notion of quality is irrelevant. If, as the writers claim, the notion of quality is indispensable, then the 'important' characteristics of the service will be the ones that have 'quality', so the definition is circular and empty.

Other definitions offered fare no better. The conception of quality defended by the great quality 'guru' Crosby, cited reverentially by Al-Assaf and Schmele (1993, p. 30), is 'conformance to requirements'. Obviously, without a clear account of what ought to be required in a given context, this tells us nothing. Joss and Kogan do not attempt to define quality as such but they do offer a purported 'definition' of Total Quality Management as:

> *'an integrated, corporately-led programme of organ-*
> *isational change designed to engender and sustain*
> *a culture of continuous improvement based on*
> *customer-oriented definitions of quality.' (Joss and*
> *Kogan 1995, p. 13)*

This tells us what we knew already: that the aim of TQM is to create a certain type of 'culture' within an organisation, via the imposition of certain practices by management which will, in some as yet unspecified way, improve the organisation. Clearly the phrase 'based on customer-oriented definitions of quality' is key to understanding the authors' meaning, although the definition does not explain their conception of quality, nor does it indicate why the concept is treated as somehow basic to evaluation. Yet again, the only substance to the concept of 'quality' appears to be that certain people (again identified as 'customers') are prepared to *say* that a thing has quality.

Persuasive definition

What is really going on in all this is not a serious attempt to define quality at all: not, at least, in the ordinary sense of 'definition' in which one explains what a term means. Rather, what is happening is something more like the process which the philosopher CL Stevenson described as 'persuasive definition' (Stevenson 1944, p. 222). Persuasive definition is possible because many terms have two elements to their meaning: a descriptive (or factual) element and what Stevenson called an emotive (or evaluative) element. The emotive meaning of a term carries a certain force: it affects our attitudes, causing us to approve (or disapprove) of whatever it is applied to, and hence it affects our behaviour. For example, the word 'democracy' has for many years had an emotive aspect to its meaning and the result is that if a government can convince us that it is democratic then we are more likely to accept it and to acquiesce under its rule than if we think it undemocratic. Persuasive definitions can take over when the descriptive meaning of a term becomes vague and unclear, but it continues to carry emotive force. To define a term persuasively is to offer as an 'explanation' of the meaning of an emotive term what is in fact a proposal for a revision of that term's descriptive meaning. If you succeed in defining a term in this way then you have persuaded the person who hears your definition to accept a revised factual significance for the term in question, but since the term still carries emotive force you have (disturbingly enough) managed to change their behaviour without, in all probability, their ever understanding the process that has just taken place (and very possibly without your fully understanding what has happened either).

The word 'democracy' is a classic example of a term that has been subject to persuasive definitions: its descriptive meaning has become vague enough for leaders and political systems of radically different types and colourings to all claim that they, and they alone, are 'truly' democratic. The descriptive meaning of the term 'quality' is vaguer still, while its emotive force is as strong as ever: who can disagree with the claim that quality is important or that it matters? So the defenders of the 'quality revolution' are onto a winner: by continually describing certain products or practices as 'demonstrating quality' they can create an atmosphere in which it seems unreasonable to question or criticise, or to deny that there have been massive improvements since the times before quality was 'rediscovered'.

This is what the business gurus have achieved: a way of labelling products as 'quality' so as to get people to buy them. No wonder senior managers and the government find the idea of applying this technique to the health service 'attractive'. Ideally, they can get everyone to accept the decisions they make simply by choosing the right terminology.

How else can we understand what is happening today, in our health services and elsewhere? The fact that so many supposedly intelligent people can talk so much nonsense for so long certainly requires some explaining. Kelly and Swift (1991, p. 26) recommend that managers be assessed 'on the basis of at least one objective which focused *exclusively* on quality'. It hardly takes great philosophical acumen to realise that it is impossible, whatever one is doing, to focus exclusively on quality. When a violinist thinks about how to improve her playing, she is not thinking about the 'quality' of the playing *as opposed* to the tone production, phrasing and any other feature of the playing apart from the quality. Rather, she is thinking about how she could do these things better and if she succeeds then she has improved the quality of her playing in the only meaningful sense of the word. The same writers explain that their Health Board, having appointed several full- or part-time unit quality co-ordinators and set up a senior management steering group, then organised a series of workshops to investigate what quality management means (ibid, p. 27). Do we really go all that way in pursuing a policy before trying to find out what that policy *means*? Similarly Joss and Kogan (1995, p. 43) admit that the TQM approach was 'launched' before being 'fully conceptualised' and they comment (ibid, p. 5) that: 'The quest for quality is made more testing by the difficulty of defining it' (which they never do). Again, we need to ask why, if they do not know what 'quality' is, they have embarked upon a 'quest' for it? How will they know when they have found it? Does one really write a book called *Advancing Quality* only to admit that one does not know what 'quality' is? Is there not something bizarre about an approach which is 'launched' before being 'fully conceptualised', especially when that approach purports to usher in a new 'culture', transforming the practice of everyone in the service?

What is particularly disturbing about this vacuous debate on quality is that it is hardly out of place in contemporary discussions of health service policy: or indeed of economic policy, education policy and a host of other issues vital to the well-being of humanity. The intellectual environment of administrators, managers and policy makers (all those people who make decisions on our behalf, with which we all have to live) is populated increasingly by such ethereal entities as missions and quality continua, who behave in a variety of bizarre ways: for instance, they 'gradually seep into the consciousness of organisations' (Hill *et al.* 1990, p. 5). The recipe for success is an articulated mission statement, the affirmation that one's commitment to quality is total and, most importantly, the ability to set oneself 'realistic' standards, meaning ones that you know in advance you can meet. The dominant ethos seems to be that by redescribing reality we can change it: by employing people to devise new ways of thinking and talking about the world we can avoid all the grubby problems that resulted from our old, outdated and defeatist views. Qualispeak is as Orwellian as Oceania Newspeak.

'The quality initiative' report celebrates 'the new and rapidly expanding vocabulary of health services management', welcoming the term 'excellence' into the fold (Hill *et al.* 1990). Services may be contracting, resources may be shrinking, jobs may be disappearing, but the management vocabulary of the health service is bigger than ever, increasing all the time, and we may be forgiven for surmising that there is a fairly direct correlation between these phenomena.

Chapter 4

The pseudo-science of management

In addition to the claim that 'quality' is somehow foundational to evaluation, such that to improve a service means to increase or improve its quality, we have seen that a key claim of management theory is that there are 'basic organisational criteria' common to all complex organisations (Berwick 1993, IHSM 1993, Laffel and Blumenthal 1993, Peters 1992). The existence of these common organisational criteria provides the basis for the claim that management is a science, a specific discipline with its own distinctive methods and principles, such that theories developed for the manufacturing sector (about how to introduce 'quality' into such process such as the production of video cassette recorders or packets of cornflakes) can mean-ingfully be applied to the project of improving such radically different practices as healthcare and education. These basic criteria are sometimes equated with the 'values' which 'under-pin' health service activity or (in specifically British writing on the application of management theory to health) the 'value-base' of the NHS. It seems that until we understand these basic 'criteria' or 'values' we cannot understand the 'purpose' of the health service but when we do understand them we acquire a special insight into the nature of the organisation and we can speak with 'objectivity' (IHSM 1993, p. 6) and 'particular authority' (ibid, p. 8) about it. The 'incorporation' of these criteria into the 'processes' of an organisation is a prerequisite for organisational success (Joss and Kogan 1995, Laffel and Blumenthal 1993) such that the health service will only become a 'coherent organisation' when it:

'is able to incorporate these [criteria] into the specific values and criteria that underpin the health service.'
(IHSM 1993, p. 23)

Unfortunately, the authors of the report which makes this claim do not go into very great detail as to what these basic organisational criteria are. Shortly after this statement, in a set of claims presumably meant to explain the criteria, they state that the purpose of the organisation must be 'clear and understood' and its values should be 'agreed'. They add that 'corporate objectives can be set . . . from the values and purpose' and that there should be a 'system of measuring the achievement of corporate objectives'. 'Accountability' and 'efficiency and effectiveness' (which are also frequently described as 'values') appear to be criteria, as do the need for a 'consumer focus' and for the organisation to be 'integrated' (ibid, p. 24). Joss and Kogan (1995, p. 53) list the following 'basic criteria' for evaluating 'TQM implementation':

- dynamic and sustained senior management commitment to TQM
- integrated planning for operations and quality at all levels
- methods and systems for systematic[10] measurement and evaluation of quality improvement
- organisational structures for quality improvement to ensure accountability for quality and support for staff in their quality improvement efforts
- education and training for staff in quality improvement methods to create a highly skilled and motivated workforce
- staff empowerment to enable the maximum contribution of all staff to continuous improvement
- movement towards a common definition of quality based on consumer requirements
- an organisational culture of continuous quality improvement.

They then state that these 'features' should be 'translated by an organisation into measurable objectives with associated measures and action plans'. They do not, however, have anything terribly precise to say to assist in the process of translating these mantra-like phrases into concrete objectives. Instead, managers are advised to bring in 'outside experts' who can 'bring a broader and more objective perspective to the implementation'. There are problems here akin to those already noted for certain theories in applied ethics (Chapter 1). Even though we may have serious differences on many moral questions, we could (perhaps) all agree on certain 'basic moral principles' – but only if they were spelled out in terms so abstract as to be platitudinous. Yet when the principles are spelled out in such terms it is obviously impossible to deduce any clear practical consequences from them, so it is not clear that they can play any substantial role in the resolution of real problems.

Since all of the Joss and Kogan 'criteria' refer to 'quality', 'quality improvement' or 'continuous (quality) improvement', until we have a more concrete understanding of these terms the criteria have very little semantic content. (Insofar as they do give these concepts any content it is via the notion of a 'consumer' – a point to which we must return shortly.) What content these phrases do have independently of the 'continuous' appeal to 'quality' is hardly very substantial. For instance, I think we can all agree that a 'highly skilled and motivated workforce' is likely to be better than a demotivated workforce with few skills: we do not really need an expert in organisational science to point this out to us. It would be more useful for the 'experts' to explain the precise nature of the 'education and training' required to achieve this high level of skill and motivation. What sort of advice would the 'outside expert' be able to give on this point and what would be the basis for his claim to be an 'expert' on the organisation of our particular practices? Why is his advice thought superior to that of someone with extensive experience of the specific context of this organisation?

If the very fact that he is from 'outside' the organisation is meant to guarantee his 'objectivity' then the reasoning behind this conclusion is obviously flawed. I have never been involved with the management of a football club, at any level, but it does not follow that I am therefore particularly well qualified to lead the England team into the next World Cup, by virtue of my 'objectivity'.[11] Presumably, then, in addition to being from 'outside', the expert's qualifications to comment on an unfamiliar organisation derive from his general expertise in management, meaning his knowledge of the general principles of good organisation which can be applied to any new practice he is charged to 'organise'. But now we have come full circle. If there really are any substantial principles of good management then this would surely be the right place for the authors to state them: in the context of a work supposedly explaining the 'theory' behind their approach to management. But if all that they can say about what an 'expert' on the general principles of good management knows is stated in their 'basic criteria', then we have been given no grounds to accept the claim that the 'expert' knows better than anyone else how to interpret and 'implement' these abstract criteria in the context of any specific organisation.

Let us suppose (purely for the sake of argument, of course) that the processes of 'education and training' envisaged by the 'expert' involve subjecting the workforce to continuous monitoring and frequent time-consuming 'staff development' exercises to 'raise' their 'awareness' about their corporate identity. From the 'subjective' perspectives of many workers 'educated' in this manner the 'skills' likely to be 'developed' will be in the filling out of forms and the cynical repetition of management jargon where required. How 'motivating' and 'empowering' these experiences are likely to be is a matter for debate. (Perhaps the reader can consult her own experience.) It is by no means clear why the 'outside expert' should speak with particular authority on this.

Spurious objectivity

Similarly, we might agree that in some sense of the words, 'accountability' and 'efficiency' are good things, which is perhaps all that is meant by the claim that they are 'values'. I say 'in some sense' because until we know precisely what a person means by either of these terms we would be foolish to accept that they are unequivocally good things. What conception of 'costs' and 'benefits' underlies a specific view of 'efficiency'? What precise mechanisms are envisaged for making people 'accountable' and who will be accountable to whom? Will the implementation of these mechanisms make for more or less efficiency? Without a detailed account of how to apply these 'criteria' in real contexts it is impossible to say, so it is impossible to know what the claim that these terms denote 'values' really means. It hardly represents the 'important contribution' which its authors claim to have made (IHSM 1993, p. 5). While repeatedly advocating 'transparency', the IHSM document offers an account of the 'values' it wants to see clearly 'demonstrated' which is hopelessly opaque. One of the few genuinely substantial (if unsubstantiated) claims of the report is that the NHS should no longer be funded by 'general taxation' (ibid, p. 39) and that other forms of funding, including private insurance and 'top-up payments', could provide a 'more effective market' (ibid, p. 42). One of the alleged advantages of these alternative methods of funding is that they would supposedly make 'the rationing process' (which the report views as an essential feature of any developed health service) more 'equitable'. But for this claim to be defensible, we evidently require a coherent conception of equity. The report at one point seems to suggest that 'equity' means 'equal care for equal need' (p. 14), although it does not explain how needs are identified and measured, so it is unclear as to how we are to know when needs are 'equal'. Without such knowledge it is obviously not possible for any rationing process to be both 'transparent' and 'based on' this conception of 'equity'.

Nor do the authors seem entirely sure that the service should be 'based on' such a 'value' since they go on to admit that there may be 'some scepticism about the legitimacy of these values' and to express the worry that this definition of equity 'violates the principle of equality' because 'some individuals derive greater benefits from the system while paying less for it'. Unlike socialist conceptions of 'equality', this 'principle of equality' appears to be concerned with people getting no more and no less than they *pay for*. The authors do not say what weight, if any, they give to the 'principle of equality', having mentioned it, nor do they explain why anyone should take it seriously as a moral principle. They do not say anything to combat the 'scepticism', either, but it nonetheless vanishes almost as soon as it has been stated, so it does not prevent the authors from confidently asserting the fundamental nature of these and several other 'underlying values' throughout the rest of the report and claiming that in doing so they have 'brought clarity to bear' on the values and purpose of the NHS (p. 44).

In addition to 'efficiency and effectiveness' (perhaps in explanation of one or both of them) the report also states that health services 'should be delivered at the highest possible level of quality' which means 'keeping to certain standards' and 'also means that the needs of the patient determine the system and not the other way around' (p. 38). Without any account of what the standards are or how one rationally sets them, and without any coherent account of 'need', these statements are vacuous. Equally vacuous is the claim that:

> 'It is axiomatic that this society should provide comprehensive healthcare to the level it is willing to afford.' (p. 39)

It is hard enough to determine what a society can afford, let alone what it is 'willing to' afford. Outside the linguistic laboratory of contemporary management literature, where the abuse of language is commonplace and where new, meaningless (and frequently horrifying) hybrid expressions are constantly being created, one would only speak of someone's being 'willing to' afford something ironically. In response to my claim that I cannot afford something, you may suggest I am not willing to afford it, to imply that it is not really a matter of what I can afford: rather I am simply unwilling to pay for something and pretending that I am unable to pay for it. So this 'axiom' states that 'this society' should pay for as much healthcare as it is willing to pay for. It does not, of course, state how much healthcare this society should be willing to pay for, so the 'axiom' states nothing: certainly nothing follows from so empty a claim. Since there is little point in having an 'axiom' from which nothing can be deduced, we can only assume that the use of such a word is part of the attempt to convey a bogus 'scientific' feeling to the proceedings, as if the authors were engaged in an enterprise comparable to Euclid's work in geometry. (As we will see, this is in keeping with the misconceived view of scientific thinking which characterises management theory. Insofar as such theorists think that they have any foundation for their 'science' it is because they mistakenly believe they can deduce substantial and general conclusions about good practice from the grammatical properties of the word 'quality'.) Equally, it is hard to find any meaning for the word 'comprehensive' in this context when the authors go to such lengths to stress that rationing is inevitable and that many services which people might desire simply cannot be provided. Despite this, 'comprehensiveness' is stated as another of the 'values' on which the service should be 'based' (p. 14).

Thus, while the report has much to say on the nature of value, very little of this is helpful and much of it is incoherent. According to the IHSM, values are things that:

- 'operate at a number of levels within the decision making process' and can 'cover the total provision of healthcare'
- 'embrace concepts' such as 'distributive justice, utility, rights, altruism and economic rationality'
- 'provide the theoretical framework for social organisations'
- may 'take on the mantle of moral imperatives' but 'in practice . . . change over time and are relative'
- must be 'agreed' or else 'every decision made would be essentially an arbitrary one'
- can 'underpin' institutions like the health service, but which
- are themselves 'based on' institutions like 'the welfare state'.

All of these claims about values are taken from the *same page* of the report (IHSM 1993, p. 14) but the same or similar claims are repeated with great frequency throughout the document and readers familiar with management theory generally will recognise the style, if not the specific content, of such claims. At several points 'values' are equated with 'principles' (e.g. 'The values that underpin the NHS are its founding principles' – p. 7) while at other points the word 'values' is used interchangeably with the word 'criteria' (such as in the discussion of 'basic organisational criteria' – pp. 23–5). We are told that values must be 'shared' if 'effectiveness' (itself stated as a 'value') is to be possible for an organisation (p. 25). (So it seems that 'effectiveness' is both that which is facilitated by the 'basic values' and is one of these values itself.) Values are at some points apparently equated with 'interests' which may conflict with one another (e.g. p. 17) while at other points it is the existence of 'organisational values' ('efficiency', 'effectiveness', etc.) which are 'broadly understood and shared by all the participants' (p. 21) that is claimed to be essential for resolving conflicts between competing interests. It is, of course, not explained how values can both be (competing) interests and at the same time be 'shared' by competing interest groups and used to arbitrate between competing interests. Nor does the report explain how values can be the same things as both 'principles' and 'criteria'. We are not told what it means to speak of a value operating at a number of levels in a decision making process or embracing a concept (one imagines some sort of reunion in the jungle, with Efficiency saying 'Ah, Economic Rationality, I presume') and we are of course given no analysis whatsoever of the various 'concepts' which the values 'embrace'.

How do values 'provide' theoretical frameworks? How do they manage (in the same page) both to be the basis for, and be based on, institutions? How is it possible for the IHSM to advocate certain values as the correct ones, on which the delivery of healthcare 'should' be based and to which we all (whatever our 'perspective') must 'agree', while at the same time declaring (without, of course, any argument) that all values are 'relative'? The report does not tell us, but it does say that values 'must be defined as realistically as possible' and that 'the application of realism to values' means that 'greater specificity implies greater commitment' (p. 16). (The authors take frequent refuge in the use of the words 'clarity' and 'specificity' while failing to specify clearly what they mean at any point.)

In short, the report reads like a very poor student essay: it is impossible to construct any meaningful question to which it would be the answer. Yet it was compiled with the help of at least seven NHS chief executives and two senior academics, all of whom are supposed to be 'experts' on the science of management and the values of the NHS. I have referred to this report in some detail to bring out the massive confusions which result from attempting to apply the assumptions of management theory to the evaluation of practices in the health service. I must stress that this and the other documents discussed are chosen simply because they are illustrative of the genre. (As I stated in Chapter 1, the point is to demonstrate the techniques of philosophical analysis by discovering the underlying assumptions at work in the literature and the problems they create.)

The confusions in this document are inevitable because the underlying assumptions its authors make are untenable. Just as there are principles in engineering which can be applied to the building of any structure, such that if one knows how to build a supermarket one can apply the same basic principles to the building of a hospital (with the addition of some context-specific information about the requirements of the users of the building), it is assumed that if one knows how to manage a business then the same principles can be applied to the organisation of any practice. One simply needs to learn the particular 'requirements' of the new area, which in the case of healthcare means incorporating empirical data about such matters as the costs of particular types of care and about what the 'consumers' of care require. Hence the constant references to 'quality engineers', 'industrial quality management science' and associated 'technical' terminology throughout the new management literature.

Because (necessarily) every organisation needs to be organised and because it is clearly the case that some organisations are better managed than others, it seems meaningful to ask what 'good organisation' means and how it is achieved. If we can only answer that question then we will have achieved something rather exciting: a broad, technical understanding of good management which can in principle be applied to each and every complex organisation, be it a factory producing toy cars, a school, a university, a regional health authority or the health service for an entire nation. Such an understanding would seem to provide the recipe for success in any organised activity whatsoever; hence management is not only a sort of science, it is surely the most important science of all since it tells us how to do just about anything as efficiently and effectively as possible. A qualified management scientist, equipped with a general understanding of good organisational practice, can rise above the specifics of any given organisation in a way that no-one else can. Thus: 'a distinctively managerial perspective . . . is critical in its capacity to bring objectivity and is too often neglected' (p. 6).

This, presumably, is why managers are described throughout the IHSM report as 'arbitrators' between the different 'partisan' groups involved in the health service, where the groups that are partisan include 'all other groups'. Managers are the 'non-partisan guardians of the process' of decision making (p. 24).

They 'set agendas'; they 'achieve resolution of conflicting or partisan interests' (p. 23) and they:

> *'speak with particular authority about the organisation, whether the health service is achieving its purpose, how well or badly the system works and how resources can be best distributed.' (p. 8, repeated p. 31)*

This line of reasoning has an implication which might have been embarrassing to more modest authors and would appear to undermine the democratic rhetoric which characterises parts of the report. Since the report speaks for the IHSM (sentences frequently begin 'It is the view of the IHSM that . . .') and the authors state that the IHSM 'has a unique authority speak [sic] for management as a whole', it follows that the authors of the report speak definitively on the purpose of the health service, such that no-one else is qualified to challenge them on this issue. Either the authors failed to notice this implication (although the tributes they pay to their own work, particularly in the Foreword, suggest otherwise) or else they fail to see anything perverse in calling for a 'debate' on an issue (the values and purpose of the health service), only (effectively) to declare themselves the only people qualified to contribute to it. (In perhaps the most bizarre moment of the report, it is claimed that health service managers 'own the outcomes' of health service decisions (pp. 8 and 31). I have no idea what the authors might mean by this, but if I ever have any inessential organ removed on the NHS I will be sure to post it to one of the senior managers who helped compile the report.)

It does not occur to these authors, nor to any of the defenders of the approach they represent, that its problems may be *conceptual* in nature, in that the *meaningfulness* of its applications can be called into question. The analogy with engineering does not work, because what it means for a building to stand up does not change in accordance with the purposes for which it is used, but what it means for an organisation to be 'successful' does. Thus the attempt to discover what good organisation *as such* means represents a philosophical error: one cannot abstract the concept of organisation (or 'organisational quality') from the context of any specific practice and expect to say anything substantial and meaningful about it. There need be no general principles of good organisation, applicable to any and every practice. One may as well argue that since, necessarily, everything we do needs to be done, there must be general principles of 'doing' that tell us how to do anything at all well, be it sexual intercourse, riding a trick cycle, playing chess or piloting aeroplanes. A general science of doing could give us an objective understanding of the basic criteria common to all successful action, which could then be applied to all of these specific areas and the 'doing scientist' would be the most important person to have around when engaging in any activity whatsoever.

So we cannot assume that 'doing well' in healthcare can be understood in terms of concepts which also define what it is to do well in the world of commerce. Far from understanding general organisational criteria first and then (on the basis of this general understanding) claiming to know the 'purpose' of the health service, one would need to think critically about the purpose of the service first, before one could hope to say anything sensible about how to achieve that purpose.

Orwellian 'education'

Surely this seems obvious. Unfortunately not. Generally, whilst management theorists are prepared to concede that there may be problems in 'operationalising' the concepts and principles of TQM, CQI and IQMS in the context of what they call 'service industries' (Joss and Kogan 1995, p. 1) they feel confident that these problems are far from insurmountable and typically they treat them as a matter of overcoming certain 'cultural barriers' (Berwick 1993, p. 36) generated by a lack of enthusiasm, widespread ignorance or irrational resistance to change on the part of practitioners in the areas in question (Joss and Kogan 1995, Laffel and Blumenthal 1993, Merry 1993, Spiers 1994). What is required, then, is 'transformational leadership' (Curtis 1993, p. 200) to inspire 'commitment' (Merry 1993, p. 57) in the workforce by providing a 'vision that drives all action' (Curtis 1993). Management specialists are needed to subject practitioners to that brand of 'education' which is all about 'changing attitudes' with the goal of 'securing commitment and behaviour change' (Joss and Kogan 1995, p. 21). Ideally these specialists should use their 'particular authority' to speak about the 'purpose' of the organisation to 'change perceptions' and 'lead opinions' (Spiers 1994, p. 189). They should endeavour to 'manage' and 'correct' both 'public understanding' and the expectations of the workforce concerning the nature and goals of the service.

Practitioners who express scepticism about the validity of the approach are treated as having 'psychological and other needs' which require 're-educative initiatives': individuals need to be 'developed' so that 'cultures' can engage in 'dynamic self-correction' (Joss and Kogan 1995, p. 43). Using the terminology of American psychologist Abraham Maslow (1968), Merry (1993, pp. 56–7) suggests that a failure on the part of clinicians to respond positively to the introduction of 'industrial quality processes into healthcare' is symptomatic of a 'failure' to achieve 'self-actualization' and that such clinicians are 'in denial'. This echoes the view of the management 'guru' Crosby (1979, pp. 32–3) that both management and the working population must be 'awakened' then 'enlightened' by becoming 'committed' to the approach, before that population can be deemed to have reached 'maturity'.

Clearly these theorists do not consider the possibility that there could be any sound intellectual objections to their approach to management, such that 'resistance' is not necessarily evidence of psychological disorder or underdevelopment on the part of the objector. The intellectual foundations of the approach are apparently treated as self-evident, for the only problems worth discussing concern how to implement the approach and how to 'enlighten' a hitherto ignorant working population. It is somewhat remarkable that the advocates of an approach which insists that every aspect of practice should be examined in detail, evaluated and continually re-evaluated seem incapable of giving any clear explanation, let alone a sustained defence, of their own basic assumptions. It appears that they do not think that there is any need for them to do so.

How can this be? How can the exponents of the new 'management philosophy' be so totally blind to the problems of their approach, and so arrogant in their willingness to dismiss sincere and well thought out objections without even the appearance of a serious response? There are at least three, related, explanations.

First, the sheer volume of the work in the area seems to some theorists to be an argument in itself. Second, many authors in the area may be genuinely confused by the grammatical properties of the word 'quality'. They would not be alone in this. One prominent author has founded an entire metaphysic upon the precise same confusion over the precise same word. Like the founders of 'management philosophy', this person is thought of as something of a 'guru' by his thousands of followers throughout the world, who are every bit as obsessive about their own 'quality movement' as the management theorists are about theirs. (They too organise workshops and training sessions where they attempt to 'convert' the unenlightened with evangelical zeal.)

The third explanation for the shocking dogmatism of contemporary management theorists concerns the influence of ideology. I have alluded to this point before, but it is now worth looking at all three points in a little more detail.

Fashion, intolerance and witchcraft

To an unreflective person, the very fact that many people believe something is as good a reason as any to believe it also. This is how fashions come about. Unfortunately, the influence of fashion is not restricted to tastes in styles of clothing. There are academic fashions: particular styles of verbal and written expression are associated with intellectual credibility in certain circles, such that to be perceived as a 'bona fide' thinker one must learn to adopt these styles, however verbose and pretentious they may be. There are fashionable and unfashionable ideas. At the time of writing, Marxism would seem to be an unfashionable idea, because most people take it as read that Marx was wrong about the nature of social relations, without having made anything resembling a serious study of his work. In certain areas (again at the time of writing) postmodernism would seem to be a very fashionable idea, since even people who have no idea what postmodernists are saying nonetheless think that

it must be something terribly important and they try to incorporate postmodernist terminology into the language they use
wherever possible, just to show how intellectual they are.[12]

To be associated with the fashionable idea is to be deemed
trendy, interesting and up to date, while to display an interest in
the unfashionable idea is to be viewed as a curious eccentric, or
worse. Academic fashions are so obviously a threat to intelligent
debate and critical thinking that it is hard to see how anyone
could openly defend their existence, yet people will still dismiss
others for being 'out of step' with whatever it is that 'everybody
thinks' these days. The fact that we now have a political culture
in which expressions like 'on message' can be used without
causing a scandal shows how far along the road to institutiona-
lised stupidity and intellectual repression we have already
moved.

In the world of health management, TQM and associated
management philosophies are obviously in vogue. When an
approach has been popular for some time, boosted by substantial
government investment and other forms of official encourage-
ment, it can gather a momentum of its own, until there comes a
point when it just seems unreasonable to question it. Some
writers in the area celebrate the fashionableness of their
favoured theories as if it were decisive proof of their truth. So
Al-Assaf and Schmele (1993, p. 11) speak of the 'inevitable tide
that is moving swiftly through levels of management' and Wall
(1994, p. 318) takes the fact that a particular approach to
management 'draws the crowds' as an argument in its favour,
while the claim that an approach does not 'draw the crowds' is
treated as a knock-down refutation.

A particularly unreflective person is likely to view criticism of
a fashionable idea as an act of outrageous arrogance: who is this
person to go against what so many people are saying? It is as if
the sheer volume of work in the area shows that there must be
something to it. Thus Heginbotham (1994) protests that 'there is
a great deal of management theory' which has been 'successfully
applied within healthcare as in other industries'. It is of course
true that the exponents of this 'management theory' have been
'successful' in getting official backing to apply their approach to
the health service. Whether or not they have been 'successful' in
the more interesting sense, that the service is actually better

than it would otherwise have been as a result of their intervention, is surely the point at issue. Needless to say, Heginbotham
defends neither this claim nor the treatment of 'healthcare' as an
'industry': he takes these points as read. Certainly he is correct
in asserting that a great deal has been written on the subject
(though on the basis of what we have seen of it so far, whether
one describes this work as 'theory' also begs some philosophical
questions) and the existence of this vast literature does call for
an explanation.

The explanation need not, however, be one that asserts the
validity of 'management science'. Consider the quantity of
human energy and resources that, in an earlier age, went into
the development of methods for detecting, exposing and punish-
ing witches, who were blamed for causing plagues, for sudden,
unexpected deaths and also for crop failures and a host of natural
catastrophes. Were Heginbotham the Witchfinder General, he
might well have pointed to the numbers of witches 'successfully' caught and condemned, and the wealth of literature on the
subject, as evidence of the validity of this approach to public
health. We would immediately recognise this argument as
question begging, since the concept of witchcraft has meaning
as part of a conceptual framework which we have been given no
good reasons to accept. So the very fact that many people are
engaged in a project does not demonstrate that the project is
worthwhile or that its conceptual foundations are sound. That
they have the approval of the powers that be most certainly does
not guarantee this. Other factors, such as compatibility with the
dominant ideology of the time, may well be at work. Books like
The Textbook of Total Quality have as much claim to the title
of a work of 'science' as *Malleus Maleficarum*.[13]

Pirsig, mysticism and the referential fallacy

The second reason for the dogmatism of management science
might seem less obvious, but it is at least as important. We
have seen that the initial appeal of the term 'quality' to the

management 'gurus' and their followers lay in its emotive properties (Chapter 3). However, we also saw that persuasive definitions (which exploit the emotive potential of a term to affect our attitudes and consequently our behaviour) can take place without any of the parties involved having a clear understanding of what has happened. Thus it may well be that management theorists are sincere in their claim to have discovered something called 'quality science', the study of the general principles of 'quality management'. This claim nonetheless represents what is sometimes called a 'category mistake':[14] to make it is to place the word 'quality' in the wrong logical category. As we will see, it is to treat it as a 'naming word' when in fact it does not name anything.

We have already noted (Chapter 2) that even skilled linguistic analysts like GE Moore can commit logical fallacies. Moore was charged with the referential fallacy because he assumed that if the word 'good' has any substantial meaning, it must refer to some real property of the things we label 'good things': a property they possess over and above their other properties. He could say very little about that property: only that it was indefinable and that we knew of its existence by intuition. To get a clearer sense of what the fallacy here is and to see just how easy it is to commit, it is worth looking briefly at the work of one 20th-century author who founds an entire metaphysical position upon it.

In Pirsig's *Zen and the Art of Motorcycle Maintenance* (1988) the character of 'Phaedrus' sets out to prove that 'Quality' exists. He uses a variety of methods to establish its reality, including getting a group of students to rank a series of essays in terms of their 'Quality' (pp. 201–3). The students' judgements display a degree of uniformity, such that although they cannot say what the thing is that they have recognised in the essays, they must surely have recognised something or else what basis could they have had for their judgements? The assumption at work here appears to be that we know that a thing exists (or is real) if we can all recognise it, even if we cannot define it. Hence 'Quality' is treated as an 'undefined [and indefinable] entity' (p. 208) whose presence or absence provided the basis for the evaluative judgements of the students. Pirsig goes on to argue (p. 210) that:

'*A thing exists . . . if a world without it can't function normally. If we can show that a world without Quality functions abnormally, then we have shown that Quality exists, whether it's defined or not.*'

Phaedrus goes on to 'subtract Quality from a description of the world as we know it', to see if its absence would make any difference. Without it there would be no 'fine arts', since there would be 'no point in hanging a painting on the wall when the bare wall looks just as good'. For the same reason poetry would 'disappear' as would 'humor' since 'the difference between humor and no humor is pure Quality'. Perhaps most seriously of all for the clean-living, outdoors, all-American[15] author, 'football, baseball, games of every sort would vanish' because 'the scores would no longer be a measure of anything meaningful'. He then considers quality in the market place and the brief comments he makes seem to anticipate management theory, such that we might suspect that some of the 'gurus' had actually been influenced by his work.[16] Without Quality there would be no basis for consumer choice. Food would be bland, there would be no 'movies' or 'parties', we 'would all use public transportation' and 'wear GI shoes'. As a consequence a 'huge proportion of us would be out of work'. (Not, it would seem, people who work in public transport since their activities are obviously incapable, as far as Pirsig is concerned, of being performed well or 'with quality'.)

Interestingly, Phaedrus notes that such disciplines as 'pure science', 'philosophy and particularly logic' would be 'unchanged' (p. 211). While, it appears, it is possible to recognise differences in the quality of student essays it is not possible to recognise differences in the quality of a person's reasoning, which would seem to imply that we have no basis for saying that anyone has ever satisfactorily proved a point. Nonetheless, reflecting on his 'line of thought' Phaedrus is said to have 'decided he'd certainly proved his point . . . Quality exists'.

Having 'proved' that Quality is real, Pirsig goes on to argue that its reality cannot be accommodated within what he calls 'traditional subject-object metaphysics'. Since Quality is real, it follows that any view of the world which cannot find a place for it cannot be the correct view of the world, from which it follows that Quality is the only real thing: that is to say, that it is not only a part of the real world, it is the whole of reality. We need not concern ourselves here with what precisely this is supposed to mean, except to note that when he attempts to explain this Pirsig quickly resorts to mysticism. After a while, if we have still not understood the point, and if we still do not see that the conclusion follows, then we just need to be 'enlightened' since 'rational argument' can take us no further. What is interesting about all this for our present purposes is the remarkable similarity between Pirsig's thinking, as sketched above, and the thinking of the management theorists.

Phaedrus treats 'Quality' as a real thing which can have tangible and measurable effects on the world. Indeed, to measure the score in a game of football is to measure Quality, since without Quality the 'measure' would be 'meaningless'. It is the presence of Quality in a work of art which makes it a 'good' work of art. The absence of that property would result in the 'art' being in fact no better than a bare wall. Its absence from the market would result in measurable economic consequences, including mass unemployment. Similarly, management theorists think of quality as a thing or 'entity' (Brooks 1992, p. 18) whose 'presence' or 'absence' can have measurable effects on such things as 'costs' (Al-Assaf and Schmele 1993, pp. 3–6, Jones and Macilwaine 1991, p. 21) and 'productivity'. It is only because they treat the term 'quality' as a referring expression that they can think of quality as something susceptible to scientific analysis, capable of entering into *causal* relationships. They assume that quality is a causal agent by implying that its presence reduces costs. It is also described as an 'input', an 'outcome' and something which one can 'add' to a process; and by adding it one 'improves' – thereby, surely, causally affecting – that process (Al-Assaf and Schmele 1993, p. v, Merry 1993). Management theorists also speak of quality as being a process itself (Brooks 1992, p. 18) and as something which not only improves other things but can itself be improved (Peters 1992). So they are not sure what sort of thing the word refers to, but they at least seem agreed that it is in fact a referring expression. The word 'quality' means something because it names something. What does it name? The property 'quality', which all good things possess and all rotten things clearly lack.

That there is something wrong with this way of thinking can be seen by considering Hare's example of the difference between a 'good' and a 'bad' painting (Hare 1983, pp. 80–1). Hare is criticising the views of Moore but we can just as easily substitute the word 'quality' for 'good' since the logical error is the same in each case. We can say of two pictures that they are exactly alike in every respect except for the fact that one of them is 'signed' and the other isn't, but does it make sense to say that two paintings are exactly alike in every respect except for this one: that one of them is 'good' and the other isn't? What could that mean? Would it make sense for me to say that I just knew by intuition that one of the two was better, if each one were exactly the same as the other? Suppose I say 'ah, but they're not exactly the same, because (as an expert on quality) I can just see that one of them possesses the property of quality while the other doesn't'. Would you know what I meant? I don't think so.

Of course, if one painting were an exact replica of the other, I might make different judgements about their quality on the basis of the claim that one of them is an original (painted by a famous artist) while the other is a copy (painted by some lesser known artist). Note, though, that even in this case, I have had to point to some property other than the goodness or quality of the paintings to make sense of the judgements about them. The point is that goodness (or quality) is not just another property which the paintings can have or lack, whose presence or absence provides the basis for judgements about them. Rather, the judgement that the paintings are good or bad must be based on some *other* property of the paintings. Similarly, the uniform judgements made by Phaedrus' students when evaluating essays are in no meaningful sense 'explained' by the claim that they are based on their perception of the essays' 'Quality'. Rather (one suspects) they were already aware of the criteria for evaluating essays, such as the coherence of the arguments and the clarity of the style, and it is these features which form the basis for the evaluation, which they *expressed* by using the word 'quality'.

So when answering the question 'what is quality?' we can be easily misled by the grammatical properties of the term. It looks like a naming word (especially if, like Pirsig, we insist on giving it a capital letter every time we use it) so we can be perplexed as to what precisely it refers to and we are soon led to the view that it must be some mystical property a thing has over and above all its other properties. (Similarly, if we think of 'the average family' as a straightforward referring expression then we may be genuinely perplexed by the claim that this family has 2.4 children.) Pirsig's argument begins with the assumption that, if a word means anything, it must refer to something (since, from the outset, he treats 'Quality' as a 'thing') and from the fact that we can meaningfully employ the term in all sorts of contexts (to evaluate anything from works of art to modes of transportation) he concludes that some thing or property must exist to which this term corresponds and that the thing must be present in all of these different contexts. (Since, in principle, we could evaluate just about everything, it is perhaps not surprising that he arrives at the conclusion that Quality is literally everywhere.)

The mistake is in assuming that the term refers to anything in the first place. It doesn't. Rather, one predicates the word of something in order to recommend that thing as a good instance of its kind. The meaning of the term is a matter of its function in the language. It is impossible to reduce this evaluative (commendatory) function of language to a descriptive function:[17] I can describe a thing by referring to its various properties and I can then commend it for having those properties, but it is just a logical error to think that in commending it I must really be describing it again, referring to some other property it has, in addition to the ones I have already named and commended.

So to say something is good or has quality is, purely and simply, to commend it. This is why it seems obvious to management theorists that 'no-one is opposed to quality' (Curtis 1993, p. 191). To criticise a thing for having quality would be to make a logical error. But this is not because quality is some magical property which improves everything it touches. We don't decide to praise something because we 'discover' it has quality, but rather to say it has quality is simply to find another way of praising it. This commendatory function is the only common strand of meaning which the word possesses in every context in which it is used. And it can be used in any number of contexts, for one might approve of, and so recommend, just about anything: a meal, an organ recital or the treatment one gets while in hospital with a damaged arm. In this sense, only, one could claim to discover quality in all these things, which is just another way of saying one can commend all these things. But the criteria for the proper application of the term to any specific instance of a given kind differ radically according to context, since one's reasons for calling something a 'quality meal' (for example) need bear no resemblance to one's reasons for saying one received a 'quality service' when sick. In this sense the word means something different in each context. There cannot (logically) be any context-specific criteria for the word's use that can be applied universally.

The consequences of this for management theory are very serious. By placing the word in the wrong logical category the exponents of this approach come to view quality as both a specific property and something which all organised activities have in common. Since they note that it is (as a matter of logical necessity) always good to have quality, they reason that it should be possible to evaluate all organised activities in terms of this 'property', by discovering how much of it is present in what they do or in whatever they produce (their 'processes' or 'outcomes'). Thus the search for 'common criteria' applicable to every enterprise begins. The theorists are by now convinced that it is possible to evaluate health services, and indeed any organised activity whatsoever, in terms of criteria imported from the world of commerce, where their 'quality science' was first discovered. It's just a matter of 'incorporating' these criteria into the new area. When they inevitably fail to discover any one concept of quality applicable to such radically different activities as producing standard lamps and healing the sick, instead of admitting the approach is flawed they retreat, like Pirsig, into mysticism, deciding that the entity 'quality', though still a single property, takes many forms, is 'nebulous' and often 'elusive' (Peters 1992). All the more need for further investment in 'quality science'. Failures to 'incorporate' quality into health-care practice are put down to reactionary 'resistance' from practitioners: hence the need to 'enlighten' them, to get them to 'focus positive' and to 'assure' them that only through commitment to quality will they, and indeed everyone, become 'empowered' (Curtis 1993, Joss and Kogan 1995, Merry 1993).

Disdaining philosophical analysis as 'not to our purpose' (Wall 1994, p. 318), these theorists have no mechanism to retrace their steps and to question the foundations of their thinking with intellectual rigour. So instead the doctrine takes on a quasi-religious status. (This was perhaps inevitable for a 'movement' whose founders were always referred to as 'gurus'.) Hence the constant talk of 'conversions', 'missions', 'visions' and 'enlightenment'. Curtis (1993, p. 201) advises managers to put their quality mission statement 'on the wall' and to 'live it continually, every day', to 'be obsessed with it or it will become history', to 'print it in employee handbooks, include it in memos, create sayings, mottoes or catchwords such as "Quality is job 1"; "Absolutely, positively, overnight"; "We deliver, we deliver"; "We love to fly and it shows".' Such nonsense looks increasingly like a fairly desperate attempt to use irrational persuasion to convince others, and perhaps oneself, of the credibility of an approach whose intellectual bankruptcy is apparent to anyone with even a foothold on the real world. So it is that an entire discipline (or 'framework' or 'leadership paradigm' or whatever you want to call it) is founded on a basic conceptual error: a discipline which combines bogus science with manufactured evangelical zeal, hiding its own massive confusion behind spectacular flourishes of gobbledegook.

Ideology and the 'swiftly moving tide'

There is a third explanation for the phenomenon of quality science and the intransigence of its defenders. We have seen that its resilience in the face of apparently decisive criticisms can be partially explained in terms of academic fashions: its sheer popularity amongst those who 'theorise' about management strikes many of its exponents as a decisive argument in its favour. We have also seen that the very idea that there could be a 'science' of quality represents a logical error. The claim to be able to evaluate every organised practice in terms of the same criteria, though strictly nonsensical, seems to its defenders to represent a meaningful and therefore possible project because they are confused by the grammatical properties of the word 'quality', which they effectively treat as a referring expression – a conceptual error which opens up the exciting (but illusory) possibility of evaluating every organised practice in terms of the same conceptual framework.

In a sense the third explanation is better, in that it explains (without invalidating) these preceding explanations. By this I mean that it is meaningful to ask why this particular approach should be so fashionable at this point in time. What is it that makes certain ideas 'take off', while others (perhaps equally bad) do not? Why did the 'quality revolution' turn into Al-Assaf's 'inevitable tide . . . moving swiftly through levels of management', becoming so 'main-stream' that the attempt to question it strikes its defenders as either frivolous or absurd, such that to do so is to be deemed 'out of touch' with the basic realities of life?[18] At the risk of being accused by philosophical purists of 'doing sociology', we can ask what conditions make the conclusions of the 'quality scientists' seem so desirable that they are inclined to make this particular sort of logical error, as opposed to founding some other (perhaps equally erroneous) approach on a different (possibly equally invalid) set of assumptions and arguments?

Often in linguistic philosophy, we are content to provide a detailed analysis of the conceptual errors underlying certain ways of thinking and talking about the world, and in a perfectly legitimate sense the confusions inherent in the thinking analysed are thereby explained. However, there is no need for the explanation to end there, and indeed the picture is surely incomplete unless we inquire as to why it is that certain types of confusion are prone to arise in particular contexts. What is it about the current social environment, in which thinking about the organisation of health services takes place, that produces the sort of errors we have seen to characterise the debate? To answer this question we need to look at the forces which shape the 'mind-set' of the contemporary management theorist and the policy makers who are inclined to welcome and encourage this theorist's approach to practice. An explanation at this level promises to be 'deeper' and more satisfying, in that it provides an account of the whole scene into which the other explanations fit and it also explains the relationships between them.

I have claimed at various points that the new language of management is ideologically loaded, that its popularity is linked to its compatibility with the dominant ideology of the day and hence that the struggle to impose it on a cynical working population is one with ideological dimensions. It is important to explain these points, not only because they help to explain the dogmatism of many management theorists but also because managers working in the health service may not wish to act as agents of the dominant ideology of the day and so may themselves wish to resist the swiftly moving tide of the new management thinking.

To say that a debate has ideological dimensions is to say at least this: that the parties bring to it assumptions of a fundamental nature, which affect the way that they conceptualise the subject matter under discussion. Many of these assumptions will be political and evaluative, in that they concern the nature of the social world and the moral relationships it gives rise to. For instance, to view the health service as a 'business' is to make assumptions about the nature and moral status of health service activities which are contentious and reflect a broader picture of the social world in the background. Marxists use 'ideology' to denote a system of assumptions which distorts reality and so diminishes our ability to solve problems. To say that someone is 'in the grip of' an ideology or is an 'ideologue' is to say that he is either unable or unwilling to subject his fundamental assumptions to critical attention. In this (negative) use of the term an 'ideological' mentality is the opposite of a philosophical mentality.[19] The ideologue treats his own basic assumptions as too obvious to need any clear explanation or defence. To such a person, the very fact that someone disagrees with (or even simply questions) his view is evidence that the dissenter has not understood.

We have seen that defenders of the new management philosophy do not seem prepared even to consider the possibility that scepticism about their favoured theories might be justified. If a working population does not see the obvious advantages of introducing the various forms of 'quality management' into its organisation then it needs to undergo some 'dynamic self-correction'; sceptics require 'education' to 'correct' their 'opinions'; people need to be encouraged to 'self-actualise' and so forth. The Orwellian flavour of this brand of 'education' is usually sweetened by the rhetoric of 'empowerment' and democratic declarations to the effect that we are all in it together, that change must come from everyone and be 'bottom up' as well as 'top down', (Joss and Kogan 1995, pp. 40–4) but what is absolutely clear is that the desirability of the changes advocated is never for a moment seriously questioned.

One of the most significant 'shifts' in 'perception' to result from the 'educative change' (ibid, p. 21) proposed seems quite overtly ideological in nature, although this point is of course not acknowledged and the ideological assumptions in question are certainly never defended. In order to grasp the benefits of the new management thinking, it is necessary for practitioners to undergo a 'paradigm shift' such that they conceptualise their activities in terms of the language of commercial enterprises. Carers must come to see the patient as a 'customer' or 'consumer' and to think of their fellow workers as 'internal customers' (ibid, p. 23, Al-Assaf and Schmele 1993, p. 84, Sage 1991). They must learn to construe health as a 'product' and to regard the process of caring as a 'production process' (Berwick 1993, p. 35). In short, they must learn to think of healthcare as a sort of business, governed by the same 'basic principles' and 'values' as any commercial venture. Similarly educators are supposed to view such things as 'learning' and even 'personal development' as 'products' which they 'deliver' to their students, who are the 'consumers' of education.[20]

How does the language of quality fit in? It is instructive to consider the fate of another term which enjoyed brief popularity in the British National Health Service in the early 1990s. At the time certain 'experts' in the field of health services management announced that the purpose of the health service was not simply to make people healthier. Rather, its goal was to produce 'health gains', where the discovery of the 'concept' of 'health gain' was heralded as a massive advance in thinking about health management. Two 'standing conferences' were held in its honour (funded, of course, with public money) and scores of publications and other circulated documents explored the nuances of this new 'technical term', which was declared to be 'a radical and challenging concept' (Chambers 1992, p. 11), the 'way forward' for the NHS (Eskin 1992, p. 2) and even the 'philosophical basis' for 'the activities of purchasing authorities' and 'the ultimate purpose of the NHS' (Liddle 1992a, p. 1). Like the exponents of 'quality', the defenders of 'health gain' hoped that their favoured concept could introduce 'economic rationality' to the NHS:

> *'The intervention that achieves the greatest health gain at the lowest cost would be judged to be the most efficient. In theory it should be possible to evaluate a whole range of different health interventions and compare the net costs of health gains from primary health promotion, secondary and tertiary prevention, and treatments.' (Godfrey 1992, p. 7)*

The explicit goal was to find a common 'currency' in terms of which different and apparently incommensurable activities could be quantified and evaluated to assess the 'productivity' of health services. Yet in the same articles in which such claims were made (often in the same paragraphs), authors admitted that they could not say what health gains were and that no known method existed to define or measure them. 'Research' into the concept typically took the form of highly paid administrators writing to their colleagues in other parts of the country asking them what they felt the term 'meant to them' and collating any responses received. Unsurprisingly, answers received usually made reference to the idea that 'producing health gains' had something to do with making people healthier, although it also had a lot to do with 'empowering' people, 'developing' them and so forth. Some of these pieces of 'research' are described in Loughlin (1993b).

Perhaps it will come as no great shock to the reader that the activity of translating the language of 'making people healthier' into talk of 'producing health gains' did not, in fact, produce any 'measurable benefits' to the 'consumers' of healthcare. It is also unsurprising (though nonetheless remarkable) that no-one ever undertook a study of the 'efficiency' of devoting large sums of public money to the project of 'empowering' senior administrators and so-called management theorists quite literally to 'investigate' the meaning of their own terminology. At a time when people with valuable practical and intellectual skills were being made redundant and patients were being told that the resources to meet their needs were simply not available, how could it seem so 'rational' to so many, to waste so much money in the name of 'efficiency'?

A clue can be found if we try to make sense of a comment made by one of the exponents of the 'health gain perspective', writing in an issue of *HFA 2000 News* dedicated to the concept of 'health gain'. After admitting that no-one who writes about this 'concept' seems to know what it means, Liddle (1992b, p. 13) nonetheless insists that:

> '*It is a pity to condemn such a potentially useful term without a serious attempt to give it some consistent meaning.*'

It is hard to see how Liddle could know that a term is useful without knowing what the term means, but if you do know what a term means then it must already mean something, so there is surely no need to 'give' it a meaning. To make any sense of this at all, we need to look at the word itself. Why should it strike certain people as 'potentially useful', even though they admit that they don't know what it means? Presumably, because it is a noun, such that it appears to name an 'output', 'product' or 'result' (Liddle 1992a, p. 1). Furthermore, it suggests quantification: if we talk about care as an activity aimed at producing 'health gains' then we can ask 'how many' of these gains were produced by a specific intervention, in the same way that we can ask how many cars were produced at a specific factory over a period of one year. (To return to a question raised in Chapter 2 (note 25) we could solve the problem of whether it is 'best' to spend a particular sum of money on increased mobility for a large number of elderly patients or on providing a chance of survival for a small group of very sick children, by working out how many 'health gains' were likely to be produced by each option.) The fact that the question cannot meaningfully be answered, because we have, in reality, no meaningful way to identify and measure health gains[21] (because somebody just made the word up) is beside the point: if we can get people to start talking about healthcare in this way then we can get them to start thinking of healthcare as a 'business' or 'industry'.

So why do the evangelists of the 'quality revolution' commit the referential fallacy? Why does a 'science' based on such a fallacy strike so many people as an exciting prospect? It is only because the word 'quality' looks like it refers to some 'outcome' or 'product' that it was ever attractive at all. The grammar of production and consumption requires an activity to have an 'output' which is measurable or else it cannot be conceived as something worth paying people to do. To make the health service into a business it is necessary, first, to get its management and workforce to start thinking of it as a business, which means getting them to conceptualise their activities as aimed at producing some quantifiable product which they deliver to the business's customers. To establish the ethos of business in the public services it is necessary first to establish a business language as the dominant language in terms of which management and the workforce in those services describe and evaluate everything they do. It will then be viewed as the 'proper' or 'technical' way to talk about services, while all other ways of discussing practice will come to be thought of as 'loose' or 'colloquial'. Whether or not the way to a man's heart was ever through his stomach, the route to the soul of a public service is through the mouths of those who provide and use it. Control the way they speak and you will soon have altered the way they think and once all involved with the service have had their thinking about it suitably adjusted, the very nature of the service will have changed.

Why then did the language of 'health gain' never really take off as the language of 'quality' has? I can only speculate, but I would suggest that its greatest flaw as a term is that it is (for the ideologues of 'management science') rather too specific, making direct reference to 'health'. In contrast, if the desired 'output' of health service activity is 'quality' and there already exists a developed language of 'quality' in the commercial sector, then it is possible to think of the goal of healthcare in the very same terms as one conceives of the goals of commercial enterprises. Quality is the goal of any production process, while health gains can only be made in the area of health. So 'quality' is much more effective as part of the broad project of making every aspect of professional – and eventually social – life comprehensible in terms of the same, free market, ideology.

Agents of the market: management as the 'enemy within'

Obviously, this rather begs the question as to why anyone should want to be part of such a project. Indeed, many of us do not want this. Darbyshire (1993) speaks for many working in the health service when he expresses a profound sense of 'alienation' and 'despair' as he watches the service being 'transformed into an ideologue's adventure playground'. To the 'untrained' eye, business and healthcare are as alike as engineering and aesthetics. The fact that healthcare incurs financial costs does not undermine this point, any more than the fact that paintings are physical objects suggests that art is a branch of physics. Why should we train ourselves to see the one activity as 'basically' or fundamentally the same as the other, when they appear at first glance to be so different and when the effort to see them as the same is indeed a struggle, requiring the construction of a new and unnatural language and requiring us to dismiss as misguided the instincts of those dedicated to working in the health service, who view the comparison with business as repellent? Why should we strive to force the practices of healthcare into a conceptual framework designed for competitive trade, against the resistance of many practitioners? Similarly, there are those of us working in the area of education who see the social project underway as destructive of values that are essential to our practices and indeed to the very fabric of our moral and social lives.

Consider the point about fees and 'grade inflation', made above (note 20). In the view of unfashionable academics like myself, a university education is for anyone with the capacity to benefit from it and the sense to want it. Admission to a university should therefore be based on an assessment of the candidate's ability to benefit from the proposed course of study, which requires an evaluation of her intellectual capacities in terms of consistently applied academic standards, not an examination of her bank balance.

However, in the new consumer culture universities must compete for students, which requires them to lower their standards of admission, and increasingly students pay their own fees. Add to this the fact that, for many students – understandably, given the competitive nature of life in contemporary capitalist society – their main reason for doing the degree is a desire for a formal qualification which will improve their market potential and not because they are naturally inclined to academic study. They may, indeed, feel that they have no direct interest in understanding their world and no 'feel' for the subject they study, which is simply a 'means to an end'. (Again, this is understandable given the crass consumerism which characterises the society in which they have grown up, where the value of anything is measured in terms of the direct material benefits it produces and where the love of learning for its own sake is almost universally derided.) The result is inevitable: institutions attempting to accommodate increasing numbers of students with low abilities and high expectations; furthermore, institutions that are under constant pressure to 'demonstrate quality' by 'producing' plenty of good degree passes.

This of course leads to administrations pressuring academics to admit, and then reward, applicants simply because those applicants have a secure source of funding. Yet for a degree result to be a meaningful measure of anything, it must indicate a genuine level of academic achievement. If academics bow to this latest market pressure, the first and most obvious casualties will be those students who, through their commitment and genuine enthusiasm for their subjects, manage to realise their academic potentials by producing really excellent work, only to find the award they finally receive devalued. However, it is clearly a process that can ultimately benefit no-one, for when this process eventually works itself out, when it is well known that all a degree result measures is the applicant's having paid for a degree, the qualification will be meaningless, therefore valueless, so the 'customer' will not have received 'value for money': by being made a 'product', education becomes a product not worth buying. The whole nature of the academic world is transformed and utterly devalued in the process.

With regard to the much wider question of the impact of the rise of free market ideology on our moral and social lives, it is at least worth pointing out that the moral superiority of the market as an organisational principle for entire societies can hardly be said to have been 'demonstrated' by its victories over alternative ways of life.[22] What we have seen is a power struggle and the conclusion of such a struggle does not represent a demonstration of moral superiority – any more than Man's moral superiority over all other life-forms on the planet will finally be established when he succeeds in making them all extinct.

Robert Wolff (1986) identifies the broad conceptual shift taking place in our political thinking, as the ideologues of free market capitalism urge us to reduce every aspect of human life to a market transaction. Commenting on Robert Nozick's massively influential text *Anarchy, State and Utopia*, Wolff identifies its bizarre style as its most disturbing feature. Even compensation for the victims of crime is discussed in the language of market economics, such that the level of compensation paid effectively determines the market price of the injuries suffered. Wolff brings out eloquently the dehumanising potential of this conceptual shift.

In any competition there are winners and losers. It is one thing to be competitive in specific contexts, for instance when running in a race. But capitalism treats social life itself as a competition: in the market we compete for the 'means of life'. To accept this is to accept what the conservative politician Alan Clark, in characterising his own, Thatcherite position, described as 'ruthless social Darwinism'.[23] This means that there will be winners and losers in life. We all know who the losers are. Many of us walk past them as we leave the train station or as we go through the centre of town on our way to a good night out.[24] That man lying by the side of the station wall; he looks in his seventies, but he is probably in his early forties. He is dying, largely because there is really no point in his not dying. No-one feels the need to do anything about this; not even he does any more. He is, simply, a loser. For the Americans the term 'loser' is already in common use to characterise not just people in the context of some specific activity (such as the person who has just been checkmated and so is the loser in this particular game of chess) but to characterise *persons as such*.

Pretty soon, undoubtedly, the same usage will infiltrate British conversation and thinking. Like all the most ugly features of American life we are bound to want to adopt it as our own. To me it is both absurd and obscene that an author like

Nozick can defend a social system which treats human beings in this way on the basis of the Kantian concept of 'respect for persons'. To treat a person's whole life as a 'loss' is to write off that person altogether, to dismiss his entire existence as the necessary down-side to a system that works pretty well for some of us. If anything makes people into a 'means' to an 'end' it is surely this. If you lose a game then you can withdraw from the game and continue with your life: you can put the loss into perspective and perhaps learn from it. Even if you took the game very seriously (you may be a serious competitor) you are still who you are, still a person in your own right; you still have many other things to live for. In short, it is not the 'end of the world'. But if social life as such is a competition then things are rather different. This is a game where to lose is to lose in life: to lose one's health, dignity, social status – everything. If you lose this game then it really is the end of the world: the end of your world. What can we make of a group of people who choose to treat each other in this way? Does it really make sense to call them a 'moral community'? Do they in fact have anything at all to be proud of? An impressive array of weaponry, perhaps?

Whatever the reader thinks about the moral status of capitalism, what she should not doubt is that the social project described is well underway and that the rise of consumerism in the health service is an important part of that process. However reticent they may be in acknowledging it, the very activity of labelling healthcare an 'industry' has ideological consequences which are not lost on the defenders of 'management science'. Consider the historical account given by Joss and Kogan of the rise of 'TQM thinking'. As they explain, 'scientific methods of management' developed in the light (or, perhaps more appropriately, the shadow) of 'changes in production processes' led to greater 'industrialisation' and 'automation', resulting in:

> '*a decline in the number of skilled workers who were responsible for a complete production process and an increase in employment of unskilled and semi-skilled workers carrying out high volume repetitive sub-tasks in narrow areas of production.*' (Joss and Kogan 1995, pp. 8–9)

In these circumstances the 'sense of individual ownership of quality for the final product' proved 'difficult to maintain', leading to the development of Quality Control and Quality Assurance mechanisms from which TQM eventually developed. These mechanisms functioned to replace the individual's engagement with the work that mass production had destroyed. In Marxist terminology, these mechanisms take as their starting point the conditions of alienation created by advanced capitalism.

It is hardly surprising, then, that some health service workers are expressing a sense of 'alienation' as a result of current developments. Increasingly, encounters between healthcare practitioners and patients, that might previously have been conceptualised in terms of unique and often implicit moral commitments, are instead being understood in terms of formal capitalist transactions, as the language of care is systematically replaced by the language of business (Darbyshire 1993). It is certainly the case that the reality of healthcare is changing, but the introduction of the new vocabulary is not functioning, simply, to describe those changes. It is also helping to shape the new reality. Lurking in the hollow foundations of Qualispeak are the forces of the market.

I will not, at this point, venture any further into political philosophy. For now it is simply worth noting that we are witnessing a cultural revolution that is as broad in scope as the Maoist experiment in China. The difference is that this revolution is taking place in almost every developed nation on the planet. It is being imposed from above and its defenders are prepared to offer no coherent arguments in its favour. Indeed, when challenged, they openly dismiss the very idea of rational argument as unnecessary. (*See* Wall's response to my criticisms in Chapter 6.) What we need, urgently, is an intelligent and public debate about whether we actually want or even understand the 'new world order' which our leaders (whatever their party) are so keen to foist upon us. Yet instead of instigating such a debate, organisations 'representing' both management and workers have for some years now opted to embrace the dominant ideology of the day and view their 'role' as communicating that ideology to their members to foster greater 'realism'. Consider the publication produced by the IHSM, criticised extensively above. The authors did not shy away from making politically controversial recommendations (for instance, the claim that 'general taxation' should no longer be the basis for funding the NHS) but they nonetheless stressed that it was not the business of an organisation representing the health service to comment on the 'social causes' of ill health.

> *'The purpose [of the NHS] is to redress differences in health status between individuals by addressing the effects of inequalities (in terms of levels of illness and rates of chronic disease) rather than their causes (such as unemployment or poor housing).' (IHSM 1993, p. 14)*

However, it seems that it is sometimes the business of the health service to address 'causes' of illness, for instance via 'health promotion campaigns' (ibid, p. 11) so long as those campaigns are aimed at individuals and their lifestyles rather than at government policies and social institutions. (The idea that 'individuals' should be held 'responsible' for their own health status is of course entirely compatible with free market ideology.) The vital distinction for the authors of the report does not, in fact, seem to be between 'causes' and 'effects' but between what would and what would not involve challenging the economic status quo. This stance is reactionary in the fullest sense of the word. It views the role of the health service as 'reacting, not understanding': treating problems that are there but refusing to consider how one might eliminate them whenever doing so would involve raising serious questions about the structure of the society within which the service must function. As far as the authors are concerned, such issues are simply 'beyond the remit' of a health service organisation, which (to be a responsible organisation) must work out how the service can accommodate the social order of the day and advocate changes within the service to achieve this goal.

Thus the key consideration for the 'future' of the service is how it can continue to be funded in a society that is no longer 'willing to afford' a comprehensive service delivered on the basis of need and (consequently) how to develop 'efficient' mechanisms for 'rationing' that service. As noted above, the claim that rationing will 'always' be necessary in any healthcare system is taken as read, since it is assumed to follow directly from the fact that resources are finite (ibid): in line with Adam Smith, the authors assume that demand for finite resources will always outstrip supply. But when the resources are treatments for illnesses which (the authors freely admit) may be caused by social conditions, they are only in demand for so long as society continues to make people sick. It is because it is tacitly assumed that there will always be inequality that the authors can confidently assert that there will always be far too many sick people for the health service to treat, with the result that there will always be a need for rationing and that current methods of funding will eventually become inadequate to meet demand.

What does not (of course) occur to the authors is that as self-acclaimed 'leaders' of the service their 'role' might be not to 'reassess the values' of the service in the light of changes in society, but to question the moral basis for those changes in the light of the values of the service they purport to represent. Instead of asking why it is that the richest countries in the world habitually make their people sick – so sick and in such numbers that they cannot find the resources to treat them all, even when their illnesses are terminal – the nature of the political system is to be taken as a 'given' in the debate about the future of healthcare that the IHSM claims it wants to see. The health service, on this view, is like the dole in that it is there simply to prevent the victims of poverty from dying, not to change the circumstances which threaten their lives. The position is like that of a battlefield doctor who continues to patch up the bodies brought in, but who never questions why the war is going on or whether it should be being fought at all, because that's not his job: such questions are the concern of the generals. How 'responsible' this stance is is surely a matter for debate. There is nothing 'realistic' (in any worthwhile sense of the word) in viewing the nature of the broader social reality which circumscribes our roles as somehow 'none of our business', for to do so is to treat it as effectively beyond moral criticism. It is not clear that we ought to conceive of our duties as being to meet whatever demands the social order makes upon us. At some point we have to think for ourselves about the sort of practices we want and about where the limits of our responsibilities lie.

The IHSM is by no means alone in its mentality. Recently we have seen the trade unions take it upon themselves to represent the dominant social order and the views and interests of the powers that be to their membership, rather than vice versa. (I wonder how many advertisements the reader has received for private health insurance and a union-sponsored credit card from her own trade union?) Many of my students are genuinely unaware of the unprecedented nature of their own situation: it was their own union leadership that campaigned vigorously to convince its membership to accept the government's abolition of the student grant and the imposition of tuition fees, thus abandoning the principle of free education for all with the capacity to benefit from it. This change was quite obviously and directly detrimental to the interests of the union's members, who were made substantially materially worse off because of it. Yet those who argued that the union should do what all unions are supposed to do, and represent the interests of its members, were dismissed as 'unrealistic' and 'extremists' by those within the union who represented the interests of the Labour Party. (For the most part, because they wanted careers in the Labour Party and so had to demonstrate that they could 'deliver support' for Labour policies.)

I will say a little more in Part Four about what a more adequate organisation would be like, one that could meaningfully claim to 'represent' its members, whether they work in health services management, in nursing, in the education sector or anywhere else. For now it is worth noting that, just as it is essential in anything that can meaningfully be called a free society that citizens learn to think 'beyond their roles' (Chapter 1), learning not simply what is 'relevant' to the performance of their allocated 'roles' but also to decide for themselves what counts as a relevant concern to them, so we need organisations that are prepared to think independently about the social order which circumscribes their functions, rather than taking their cue from that order as to the 'role' they should play within it. An acceptable management organisation would not represent the interests and thinking of the dominant economic order to the health service. Rather, it would represent the interests of that service to the wider social order. To express a quite deliberately 'un-American' sentiment,[25] it would ask not 'what can we, as a service, do for the broader social order?' but 'how can that order change to accommodate us?' The ideals of the NHS, such as the belief in a service which is funded by those who can afford it and provided to those who need it most, are by no means bad ideals and what most people in the service are trying to do is eminently worthwhile. If that no longer 'works' in the business-led culture of New Britain then instead of asking how the health service can change to accommodate that culture, with its conceptions of efficiency and good practice, we should perhaps instead ask what is wrong with New Britain. We need to buck the trend of groups representing capitalist ideology to the workforce to show how 'reasonable' they are and to have them pointing out instead just how unreasonable are the demands that are being made upon that workforce.

Only then could we begin to have a real debate, not about the sort of service we want, given the values of our society, but about the sort of society we want and how it can provide for us the services we need. These are essentially moral questions and they concern our most fundamental assumptions. I might have concluded by saying that we need to stand up for what we believe in, but perhaps what we need first is to think with clarity, tenacity and intellectual honesty about what, exactly, it is that we do believe. Instead of treating the dominant ideology as beyond question, we need to foster an atmosphere of critical discussion of all the assumptions that frame the current debate about healthcare. Instead of dismissing serious thinking about fundamental questions as 'not to our purpose' we need (to borrow another silly phrase from another management theorist) to make that intellectual project 'job 1'. In short, we must be prepared to do moral philosophy. To think analytically about our basic values is to do moral philosophy. The alternative, offered by the new management theorists, is to give up on critical thinking altogether; to replace it with the constant repetition of unanalysed dogma and as a consequence to talk nonsense about what matters most: the values in terms of which we are to live our professional and social lives. If anything counts as a sin it must surely be this.

In the next chapter, then, it is necessary to examine the nature of applied philosophy, before moving on (in Chapter 6) to a consideration of its limits.

Part Three

Philosophy: a course in moral and intellectual self-defence[1]

Chapter 5

The fall of philosophy . . .

In discussions of social policy, the arguments of philosophers are often all too easily dismissed by those lacking either the ability or the inclination to follow their reasoning through to its conclusions. When confronted with detailed analyses demonstrating the incoherence of their pronunciations or the irrationality of their policies, politicians, senior administrators and others in positions of power find it is usually sufficient to respond by labelling such criticisms 'abstract' or 'esoteric' and then proceeding exactly as before. The assumption, sometimes implicit, sometimes spelled out but rarely supported by argument, is that philosophy is by its nature incapable of contributing to the discussion of substantive questions. Philosophers may be 'logical' people but despite, perhaps even because of, this they are not sufficiently 'practical' to understand such 'real-life' issues as justice in healthcare and the distribution of scarce resources. Anything they have to say on such matters may therefore be declared a merely 'academic' observation and effectively ignored.

Those of us who are philosophers by training or profession would like to think that such dismissive attitudes to our discipline are entirely the product of the stupidity (natural or wilful) of those who hold them. Unfortunately the truth is not so comforting. Philosophers themselves are at least in part responsible for the misconceptions surrounding the subject. The view that philosophy has nothing to say about matters of practical importance is itself the product of a doctrine promoted enthusiastically by some of the most influential philosophers of the 20th century. Perhaps still more seriously, however, it can be argued that even those philosophers dedicated to applying philosophical methods to such questions as the organisation of healthcare assume models of reality which actually serve to distort the world they purport to analyse.

This situation is disastrous, not only because intelligent people are wasting their skills. As we have seen, a society where philosophy is derided or deemed irrelevant to practical concerns is a society unable to analyse its most fundamental assumptions and as such is an ideologue's paradise (Chapter 4). A population unable to think critically and analytically about the underlying suppositions behind the messages it receives is at the mercy of those who control the media in a very real sense, because the way that population conceives the world is determined by forces which its members fail to understand, let alone control (Chapter 1). Since the way in which we conceive the world includes our conception of the moral relationships existing between ourselves and others, it shapes the values which determine how we live our lives, so such a population can in no meaningful sense be described as in control of its own destiny and cannot plausibly be said to populate a 'free' society.

The absence of any serious philosophical component to political debate throughout the developed world is glaringly obvious. The agenda is dominated by crude appeals to self-interest and to unanalysed dogma, appeals made by those whose years of experience sitting on committees and reciting slogans in public have convinced them that these are the only elements of human thought worth evoking. The stupidity which increasingly characterises political comment is accompanied by increasing barbarism in the societies whose decisions are made in such a brutish fashion. We have noted the brutalising effect of the social project underway in every developed nation[2] and that its completion requires a 'conceptual shift' on the part of management and practitioners in all of the public services and indeed within the population as a whole. We have also seen that the character of and rationale for this conceptual shift have at no point been adequately explained, let alone defended, but rather the shift is to be imposed upon a population whose uninformed, uncritical nature is taken for granted (see Chapter 4, in particular the arguments under 'Orwellian "education"' and 'Fashion, intolerance and witchcraft'). It is by no means a coincidence that the decline in the fortunes of philosophy (and other traditional academic disciplines aimed at improving the quality and rigour of human thought) has been accompanied by the rise in the influence and status of the political 'spin doctor', whose science is the manipulation of an intellectually disempowered populace. While the relationship between the stupidity and the barbarity of a society may not be a straightforward matter of cause and effect, the failure of philosophy to influence popular thought means that one more line of defence is lost against those who would reduce every aspect of life to a brutal competition. Those philosophers who have been happy to disclaim any relationship between their methods of thinking and the concerns of real life have not only presided over a near-catastrophic decline of the subject, both in material and in intellectual terms; they have also contributed to the general intellectual decay which is the hallmark of political dialogue in all the most 'advanced' countries of the world. Fiddling while the city burns may still be wrong, even though it is not the cause of the fire.

In what follows I will bring out the philosophical assumptions that brought about the nearly terminal decline of philosophy in the dying years of the 20th century, exposing their influence upon the character of political debate in society generally and even upon the thinking of many contemporary applied philosophers. There are dangers, even, in the use of the term 'applied philosophy', which can suggest a misleading distinction between 'pure' and 'applied' branches of the subject, encouraging an overly simplistic account of what it means to 'apply' theory to practice. In the scramble to prove themselves 'useful' again, many philosophers have neglected certain questions that are fundamental to the enterprise of 'applying' their method of thinking to the social world. As a result they risk losing sight of what is absolutely essential to the nature and value of the discipline, in the process making themselves 'useful' to all the wrong people and for all the wrong purposes. Rumours of the subject's survival may alas still prove to be exaggerated.

The philosopher's suicide attempt

So pervasive is the view of philosophy just sketched that the statement that it is a misconception may well require explanation. We have seen (Chapter 1) that philosophy is characterised by its method of approaching questions and also by the sort of question that philosophers tend to raise. Those who claim that philosophy is practically irrelevant are correct in asserting that its approach is essentially a logical one. Their error is in thinking that there is some sort of opposition between the practical and the logical. Philosophers are trained to reveal the logical structure of arguments and to identify and analyse key assumptions, clarifying debates by exposing ambiguities and errors of reasoning. Far from being an alternative to practical thinking, it is essential, if thinking is to provide the basis for coherent practice, that logical confusions, about the meanings of terms and about the implications of statements, are identified in this way. We have already seen that many of the confusions in the new management thinking are determined by a failure to subject the key claims made in the area, and the key concepts employed by theorists, to this sort of analysis. The absence of a serious philosophical component to the thinking of managers threatens to make them unwitting agents of an ideologically inspired movement whose goals they may well reject, if given the chance to think clearly about the matter. This is undoubtedly why the ideologues of the new approach are so dismissive of philosophy: the very last thing you need if you want to dupe an entire professional group is the widespread practice of sustained analytical thinking on the part of your potential 'converts'. The choice, in health services management and in any area of professional and social life, is not between practical and logical thinking but between clear practical thinking and confused thinking, and only the dishonest can profit from the prevalence of confusion.

We have also noted that the characteristic style of philosophical enquiry dictates that questions of a particularly fundamental nature should constitute its typical content. In most discussions, logical analysis of the key terms used leads fairly quickly to the questioning of fundamental assumptions. For instance, when confronted with claims about what would or would not improve the efficiency of the health service, philosophers will raise questions about the concept of health itself and about the purpose of healthcare. They may also want to discuss the nature of benefit, as well as what it means to describe something as a 'cost'. This is because, on any plausible analysis of the term 'efficiency', being efficient means achieving one's ends in the least costly manner. Thus it is impossible to assess the claim that a particular policy would improve efficiency unless one knows what its ends are, why they are thought to be beneficial and which effects of the policy are to be counted as amongst its 'costs'. To give an obvious but nonetheless pertinent example: is the psychological and material damage suffered by persons deprived of employment counted as amongst the costs of 'labour-saving' policies which result in redundancies? If so, how are these costs to be incorporated into the calculation of a policy's 'efficiency', and if not, then what is the justification for employing a conception of 'cost' which ignores such social factors?

Anyone who denies the practical relevance of raising such fundamental questions is only masking her own deep confusions about them or else (perhaps more dangerously) is supposing that certain answers to these questions are just obvious and as such are in need of no support nor even explicit articulation. Philosophers are sometimes criticised for raising queries about matters too obvious to merit serious discussion and if an explanation is given for this statement it is likely to be that most people do not, in fact, discuss such matters, that there is general agreement about them. Frequently this is either false or misleading. Despite the protestations of certain 'management theorists' (Heginbotham 1994), there most certainly is not general agreement that the application of their 'distinctive' approach to the problems of organising the health service has been an unequivocal success and we have seen that where general principles are widely agreed upon it is only because they are so general as to be virtually platitudinous. (Consider the 'criteria' proposed by Joss and Kogan (1995) discussed in Chapter 4.) In public debate generally, statements which begin: 'everyone accepts that . . . ' turn out, on close examination, very often to be either vacuous or actually false.

However, even the fact that a belief is widely held clearly is not, in itself, sufficient grounds to assert its truth. The move from the claim that many people hold a certain belief to the assertion that one's audience ought to believe it also embodies one of several highly controversial philosophical assumptions about the nature of truth and its relationship with belief. It might be the assumption that the truth of a belief is somehow irrelevant to the question of whether or not one ought to believe it; that one ought simply to accept the views of the majority without question. Or it could be the assumption that the very fact that a belief is widely held is sufficient to make it true, that that is all there is to a belief's being true. Less radically, the supposition could be that wide acceptance of a belief is good, if not conclusive, evidence for its truth, since on the whole people tend to have good reasons for what they believe. If we are discussing beliefs of a fundamental nature, about the nature of health or about what sort of things are really valuable or beneficial, even this assumption is highly questionable, especially when one considers the extent to which we are subjected to irrational persuasion aimed at swaying public opinion on such matters. The assumption would only hold true in societies where people gave serious thought to fundamental questions. It can hardly, therefore, be evoked to imply that such serious thought is unnecessary and that it can satisfactorily be replaced by appeals to what people generally believe.

Thus philosophy is unavoidable in practical discussion, not only in that its methods are a necessary feature of coherent practical reasoning but also in that one cannot avoid making philosophical assumptions (meaning assumptions about the sort of fundamental questions that philosophers typically address) when discussing any substantial question whatsoever. The refusal to discuss philosophy is the intellectual equivalent of putting one's fingers in one's ears whenever one's own most cherished assumptions are subjected to questioning. This much has in fact already been established, in Chapter 1 and in the discussion of academic fashions in Chapter 4. It is worth stressing here, however, since it raises the question of philosophy's demise in contemporary society: how did such an important element to practical thinking come to be abandoned?

As hinted above, it would suit a person with my own background and predisposition to believe that philosophy was the victim of a malicious attack by those who have everything to gain from the demise of critical thinking. While there may well be something to this, it is by no means a complete and honest picture. An honest description of the decline of philosophy would note that, in the first instance at least, the rot came from within. The general perception that there is a gap between the concerns of philosophy and all non-trivial discussion derives largely from the work of professional philosophers. Logical empiricism (or positivism) was, for much of the 20th century, the dominant view amongst philosophers and even today, although most of the epistemological assumptions of the positivists have been refuted, many philosophers still accept their irrationalist account of moral thinking or some watered-down version of it.[3] Positivists denied that philosophy could play a role in any practical discussions about what ought to be done, either by individuals or by societies, not because they took a dim view of philosophy but because they viewed the practical as an arena where rationality has no role. According to this doctrine, there is no right answer to any question about what is good or about what we ought to do. Although my views about what is right or wrong in any specific instance may be affected by my views about the 'facts of the matter', the evaluative component to the meaning of moral terms expresses a purely 'subjective' reaction to those facts and that reaction is not itself susceptible to rational analysis or argument. The answers to questions about how we should live are ultimately determined by irrational (or 'non-rational') considerations, in that individuals appeal to their own, purely subjective preferences and any attempt I make to convince you that you ought to behave in a certain way must involve a large dose of emotive persuasion.

A classic statement of this position is provided by Ayer (1987, pp. 26–9 and 136–50). The point of moral argument is 'to affect another person in such a way as to bring his sentiments on a given point in accordance with one's own' (p. 28). This may be achieved by calling to his attention 'certain facts that one supposes him to have overlooked' but when that fails it is also possible 'to influence other people by a suitable choice of emotive language' (p. 29). Ayer is clear that whenever 'normative expressions of value' are used 'the question of truth or falsehood does not here arise'. Moral debate, on this view, is like a battleground where the strongest passions win out and there is no tenable distinction to be drawn between rational argument and sheer propaganda. (This is in keeping with Ayer's general view of philosophy (ibid, pp. 34–5), whose 'business' is to 'solve [linguistic] puzzles' rather than to 'discover truths'. Only empirical science can claim to discover non-trivial truths.)

The effect of this view on the atmosphere in philosophy departments is best explained with reference to an anecdote about a former professor of philosophy at Manchester University.[4] I swear that it is true. A young man comes into the departmental office wanting to find out about courses in philosophy. He has the 'good fortune' to find that the professor himself is there. The professor asks him why he wants to do the subject. He replies, with obvious enthusiasm, that philosophy has always seemed to him to be the subject which takes on the 'big questions'. He is curious about the world. He wants to understand the nature of reality. He wants to find out what it all means, whether there is any purpose to life. He wants to know how he should live and what he should believe. What is more, he wants to find out if there is any clear method for answering these questions in an intelligent way, since most of the answers he has come across seem to be based on dogma. The professor laughs out loud. 'What on Earth did you expect them to be based on? Ask a stupid question . . . Really, we don't concern ourselves with nonsense like that. In the first week you will realise that such questions are meaningless! Questions about how you should live are subjective. And if you want to know what the world "really is" then you are either asking a question which has no meaning or you need to go and talk to a scientist.' Dejected, the young man leaves, without taking any printed information on the philosophy courses available. As far as I know, he never pursues a course in philosophy. This strikes me as tragic, because his reasons for wanting to do the subject were excellent.

Under the intellectual leadership of the positivists, philosophy became the most suicidal discipline of the 20th century. Some philosophers seemed positively to revel in the total practical irrelevance of their academic interests and their self-proclaimed disdain for the irrational social world was by no means lost on those who controlled the funding for academic institutions. For many years 'ethics', the most obviously practical branch of philosophy, was either ignored or derided, such that even now, in many philosophy departments, ethics and certainly applied philosophy are still not viewed as 'proper' branches of the subject. (If applied philosophy is offered at all, it is often treated as an 'addendum', something to cater to the more 'empirically minded' students not quite up to the hard, technical aspects of the discipline. Thus it is seen as a largely 'post-philosophical' enterprise, unworthy of the sophistication and attention to detail that would be taken for granted in most other areas of philosophy. This perhaps accounts for the utter futility of some of the discussions in the area.)

Philosophy is still trying to live down the caricature it made of itself; a caricature its enemies appeal to whenever they want to dismiss it today. However, once we understand the thinking behind the view that philosophy has nothing to say about practice, we realise that this view cannot be consistently appealed to by policy makers who wish to dismiss a philosophical critique of their policies. For to do so they would have to embrace the irrationalism upon which the view depends. They would need, in short, to admit that their policies are not only rationally unjustified but in principle unjustifiable and that their decisions are not a reasoned attempt to work for something called the public good (whose nature they, with their 'practical' knowledge, understand) but rather they are simply the expression of their own non-rational preferences.

It seems clear that, whether they admit it or not, public officials do in fact assume an irrationalist account of human decision making, indicated by the fact that discussion about what is valuable, and about what makes a society a good society, is reduced in so much political debate to the invention of persuasive rhetoric and the repetition of slogans. The hope is, apparently, that one's own side's slogans will have the most emotive appeal for most people or, failing that, that the desired reactions can be generated in the audience by a sufficiently skilful use of persuasive language. For when these slogans are subjected to serious questioning there appears to be nothing underlying them, other than some gut reactions which are taken to be somehow unchallengeable.

The result is the intellectual vacuum that is contemporary political conversation; a conversation characterised not by an attempt to understand and communicate the truth but rather by the use of whatever rhetorical techniques are thought to work best, the goal of contributors being to sway the undecided towards their own, pre-established stance. So natural is this picture to those of us brought up in a liberal political culture that it may seem simply to characterise the essence of practical debate, such that the shocking stupidity of a society which makes all its most serious decisions in this way rarely troubles us. This is perhaps the greatest testimony to the success of the logical positivists: their assumptions about practical thinking have become so deeply embedded in the commonly accepted picture of the social world that they are treated as obvious by people who have never even heard of the expression 'logical positivism'. A theory has really 'made it' when it slips so far into the background that it no longer seems, to the majority of people, to be a theory at all; it is just the 'way it is'. As we will see (Part Four) even authors who view logical positivism as a doctrine 'long since discredited' are in fact influenced by its assumptions.

Reviving practical philosophy: the intellectual task

The thinking of the positivists about the irrationality of values was determined to no small extent by a set of assumptions we have already had reason to examine in some detail: the belief in the 'fact–value gap' and the view that the very existence of this 'gap' makes rational thought about value impossible. While 'factual' claims are 'objective' because they can be empirically verified, value-judgements must be supplied by subjects and so are mere expressions of subjective preference. The assumptions at work here have already been refuted (see Chapter 2, under the heading 'Facts and values'). The claims that a subject needs to 'supply' a reaction to any set of facts in order to evaluate them, and that this reaction is not 'entailed' by a description of those facts, may be true but they do not show that reactions cannot be judged more or less rational or that they are simply expressions of preference. The evidence we have for any assertion (whether it is a 'factual' or an 'evaluative' claim) does not logically entail the assertion but this does not mean it cannot provide us with a good reason to believe it or that the assertion simply expresses a preference on the part of whoever utters it. If it did, then every claim we make, even supposedly factual ones, would be mere expressions of preference.

What we need, then, is a defensible theory of rationality. We need to know how to identify good reasons in practical contexts and to analyse the different types of concern that are relevant in any given situation. The moral theories considered so far (Chapter 2) were helpful in distinguishing different broad categories of 'reason for action', but none of them represented a full and satisfactory account. The reader has been warned that a philosophical approach to practical problems – in contrast to various 'quick-fix' approaches which promise much but deliver nothing of substance – requires patience and tenacity. It is sometimes necessary to retrace one's steps, to look at an issue from a variety of angles. There are a number of techniques one has to master to think philosophically. (For instance, in the discussion of moral theories it was necessary to step back from the debate to consider its *form*, in order to see what common assumptions the various parties were making.) An essay title I set for my undergraduate ethics students is: 'Write a sustained philosophical critique of your most deeply held moral belief'. It is important that we learn how to distance ourselves from even our most fundamental assumptions, to see the world from perspectives radically different from our own, to get a real sense of the appeal of positions we reject. Only then can we claim to have understood those positions and, if we still want to reject them, to have good grounds for doing so. To attempt to think in this way is to aspire to becoming a reflective person. (It is easy to spot the students who 'cheat' by using the essay as an excuse to attack a position which they in fact oppose. They are the ones who gain nothing from the exercise.)[5]

Now, having argued that the irrationalism of the positivists is false, it does not follow that we should necessarily despatch this position to the waste-bin of refuted ideas and move on, giving it no further thought. It is as foolish to ignore the history of ideas as it is to ignore the lessons of history generally. The very fact that this philosophy exerted such power over some of the finest minds of the 20th century suggests that it must have had some features to recommend it. It is worth thinking about what those features might be before attempting to construct an alternative view about rationality. Therefore, in what remains of Chapter 5, I want to look at why irrationalism seemed so appealing to so many people and why it still does appeal to many who study philosophy. There is much that needs to be preserved in its critique of certain views which may be labelled 'rationalist'. In certain respects the irrationalists had a better sense of the nature of social reality than some contemporary bioethicists. By looking at what is right in irrationalism, without thereby embracing it, I hope to develop a defensible conception of rationality which can then be applied to the question of how to reason in the context of an irrational and often brutal social world. I shall argue that the considerations which make the irrationalist view attractive do not in fact establish its truth. On the contrary, they provide reasons to search for an account of moral thinking compatible with the view that there are good and bad ways to argue about ethics and that the truth about how we ought to treat one another can sometimes be discovered. A fuller picture will emerge in Part Four, but the ensuing inquiry is necessary to prepare the ground.

Trivialising morality

Despite the celebrated demise of logical positivism in philosophical circles, many people (including many philosophers) are still attracted to the view that rationality and morals have nothing to do with one another: the claim that ethical disputes are 'a matter of opinion' is very common and is apparently taken as read by many non-philosophers. It is at least appealed to whenever people are asked to give a rational defence of some moral claim they have made and find that doing so proves difficult. The retreat into irrationalism makes my moral opinions my own private property and so immune from criticism – hence the claim that I am 'entitled' to my opinions, however stupid and indefensible they may be. The price paid for this protection, of course, is that I am no longer able to convince anyone who happens to feel differently that they really ought to agree. Moral beliefs are relegated to the status of a hobby: they are things we say to fill the silences between eating and sleep, but nothing we need take so seriously as to fall out over. It is somewhat ironic that a view about morals which grounds them in the way we feel often has the practical consequence of relegating moral beliefs to a status akin to mere tastes, such that we cease to feel so strongly about them.

Hence well-educated liberal subjectivists can 'agree to disagree' about whether it is wrong for the West to impose its vision of civilisation on the world by incinerating civilians in air raid shelters and on buses and poisoning the environment for the future generations it purports to be 'liberating'.[6] Far from being a model of civilisation, such a society is one which treats the rest of the world as mere images on a screen: for if such things are not worth falling out over then what, precisely, is there that merits an 'extreme' reaction? (If I come around to your house one day and shoot your dog, do you see this as a reason not to invite me back for dinner soon? If not, what does this show about your claim to have 'really cared' about the animal?) Yet it is against this background of utter complacency, this trivialising of morality within contemporary liberal society, that the very subjectivist assumptions which (in fact) give rise to it can seem plausible.

Many students of philosophy are attracted to irrationalist (or 'subjectivist')[7] accounts of moral thinking because they seem to provide the most realistic account of how moral arguments are framed. Moral discourse most often does resemble a verbal battlefield where people use any tactics at their disposal to sway others round to their opinion. The description of contemporary moral and political debate given in CL Stevenson's anti-rationalist classic *Ethics and Language* (Stevenson 1944) is perhaps the best in existence and I have argued (Chapter 3) that his analysis of the use of persuasive language accurately describes very much of the discussion taking place in health services management today. For these reasons Stevenson's picture may 'ring true' but we should not confuse a good description of moral and political argument, as it is conducted at a particular time in a particular culture, with an account of the essential nature of all practical thinking, as it is and must be for all time.

It is perhaps fair to point out that Stevenson would probably resent being associated with the claim that 'there is no distinction between moral argument and sheer propaganda'. He would undoubtedly disapprove of many of the more unpleasant uses of propaganda which we have seen in recent history, particularly those which sway people by means of straightforward deceit. The point is that his objections to such forms of argument would surely be moral, rather than logical, and on his own emotivist analysis his moral views should surely be analysed as expressions of his personal emotive reactions, no more true than anyone else's. Stevenson's picture (like Ayer's) does allow a role for rationality in moral arguments, in that much moral argument concerns pointing out inconsistencies and exposing the fact that the reasons given for certain attitudes involve appeals to (empirically) false beliefs. However, given that there seem to be no logical limits on what sort of beliefs can provide reasons for specific attitudes, it is not clear how I can be criticised if, when you point out that the claims I have made in order to justify my attitudes are false, I accept your statement but do not change my attitudes: your argument has simply failed to convince me. You might criticise me morally for my failure to alter my attitudes but you could do that anyway, simply for holding attitudes different from yours, and similarly I could criticise you. The point is that neither of us, on this view, could be said really to be right.

To see what is missing from Stevenson's analysis, it is worth considering an analogy with a game of football. For reasons which will become apparent, I have picked the worst football match which I personally can recall watching: the 1990 World Cup Final between Argentina and West Germany. Suppose an alien being had visited the planet Earth at that time and watched the match. What might it conclude about the game of football? It might well conclude that the game is characterised by certain key features: players attempt to render the other side ineffective either by physically injuring them or by convincing an individual called 'the referee' that members of the opposing team are guilty of attempting to inflict injuries on one's own side. The more times you deceive the referee, either by injuring an opponent without his noticing or by convincing him that a collision with an opponent was the result of an intentional and vicious attack, the better you are doing. The more pain you inflict on your opponents the less able they are to compete with you and every time you convince the referee that the other side's violence has left you in unbearable agony, you are rewarded with something called a free kick and perhaps, if your display of suffering is very convincing, the referee waves his red card at one of your enemies, who is then removed from the game altogether. The alien might reasonably conclude that football is a game which has no use for skill nor for the intelligent application of tactical thinking: the role of the manager might well appear to be largely ornamental, due to the lack of any discernible collective strategy employed by the teams. Given that this match was broadcast all around the globe, the alien might be forgiven for thinking it representative. More importantly, it would not matter if it *were* representative of how professional footballers typically play the game: this would still not imply that the alien had understood the game's essential nature, because there is no need to play football in this way and because, in fact, this is how football *should not be* played. The alien could not be said to have fully understood what it saw until it recognised that what it witnessed was a *bad* game.

Similarly, Stevenson's description of methods of argument in modern Western society may be an accurate description of public debate, simply because the standard of debate is typically very poor. It may well be, as MacIntyre (1981) claims, that we have forgotten how to argue properly or, more simply, that we often do not argue very well. Certainly, the displays of sophistry and verbal jousting provided by our political leaders and regularly beamed into our homes in the guise of political dialogue set us an example of practical thinking as poor as the lesson in sportsmanship offered by the thugs and poseurs of the 1990 World Cup Final.[8] Stevenson's account seems less plausible when we realise that it implies there is nothing *wrong* with such methods of argument; that, for example, there is nothing illogical about describing a service which spends ever more money on highly paid administrators, while making skilled carers redundant, as thereby exhibiting 'total quality'.

Until you understand that there is a distinction between good and bad arguments, there is something missing from your account of our common conception of what an argument is. To give an empirically based account of the logic of moral discourse is to assume that there are no irreducible evaluative concepts that one must apply *before* one can be said to understand what morality is. Stevenson's position would seem logically to imply that our only conception of a good argument would be one which in fact did convince people and similarly, a bad one could only be an argument which failed to convince. But it is part of our concept of a rational agent that he or she is convinced only by good arguments and is convinced by them *because* they are good: we cannot, therefore, say that arguments are good by virtue of the fact that they convince people, without vicious circularity.

We may have further reason to doubt that accounts of moral discourse based on an analysis of contemporary debates represent the right theory about ethics as such, when we realise that the nature of moral argument in our culture is to some extent determined by the dominance of the same theory whose plausibility it is being used to defend. The influence of subjectivism in ethics goes back even before (and indeed well before) 20th-century forms of positivism. The philosophical and economic theories which helped to shape the intellectual culture of Western society were massively influenced by subjectivist assumptions, so it is no surprise that the conversations of persons within that culture seem to reflect those assumptions.

Moral psychology: feelings, reason and motivation

Even so, subjectivist ethics do have an independent appeal since they stress the role of feelings in the formation of moral attitudes. Perhaps the most compelling defence of subjectivism is found in the work of David Hume and it is his account which provides one of the clearest statements of the irrationalist position on the relationship between reason and feeling. Reason, he claims, can under no circumstances motivate: only 'the passions' can do this. If morality were only about reasoning then it would have no influence over human action, instead of exerting the enormous influence which in fact it does (Hume

1989, pp. 455–7). This certainly rings true: we don't deduce or infer the wrongness of torture, we *feel* that such things are wrong (pp. 470–1). However, it is a long way from this observation to the assertion that all there is to something's being wrong is our feeling that it is wrong. (As noted above, if that is what we think, then we are actually less likely to feel strongly that the thing is wrong.) Hume's view on the relationship between feeling, reasoning and action seems to be straightforwardly causal. On this view both our beliefs and our attitudes are the causal product of non-rational factors, either biological or cultural, and our feelings motivate us by causing us to act in certain ways (ibid, pp. 470–5). For instance, if I am so constituted that I abhor violence then I will view violence as wrong and this will cause me to avoid violent behaviour. The role of reason in action is to 'serve' my feelings by telling me how to act in order to achieve my end of avoiding violence. Similarly, if I happen to like violence, then the role of reason would apparently be to tell me how to seek out as many violent situations as possible.

Hume's concept of the feelings or passions is overly simplistic and thus the view which it determines of the relationship between attitudes, beliefs and behaviour is somewhat misleading. He claims that the distinction between tastes, things we simply like or dislike, and more sophisticated types of feeling, such as emotions or attitudes, is simply a matter of the subjective quality of the experiences in question: things just 'affect' us in different ways, arousing qualitatively different responses (ibid, pp. 471–2). I dislike peanut butter, I dislike the music of The Prodigy[9] and I dislike people being tortured. It is the specific nature and intensity of my dislike in the case of people being tortured that makes this a 'moral' response. The correct view would seem to be that these categories represent logically very different types of thing altogether. If asked why I dislike the taste of peanut butter, it makes sense for me to say that I just do and no matter how intense my dislike for it, the explanation that this is just the way I feel will suffice. On the other hand, suppose I have an emotion such as fear. Emotions presuppose beliefs: if I am afraid of something then it follows, logically, that I believe that the thing I fear can harm me. It is this belief (or, rather, the truth of this belief) which provides me with a good reason to fear something.

This is why we can be criticised for having irrational fears. To give an obvious example, insects are a threat to hygiene but for many people their fear of particular insects is out of all proportion to the potential for harm which these creatures possess, and such people are rightly labelled irrational. This criticism would not even be meaningful if emotions were logically on a par with tastes, such as the preference not to eat peanut butter, which are logically beyond criticism since they require no reasons. Suppose someone feared peanut butter: when asked why, it would not do to say that he just did. This fear is so bizarre that it would require special explanation: we might perhaps search for the incident in his life which led him to associate this food with something harmful. (Perhaps he was force-fed with it as a child.) What we would not say is: that's just the way he feels, and be satisfied with that explanation.

It is also true that emotions have logical links with behaviour, such that my claim to fear something can be questioned by observation of my behaviour. If I claimed to be terrified of spiders but did not seem the least bit worried when one began to crawl up my arm, this would require some explanation. I might be said, for instance, to be exercising enormous self-control, perhaps because I am embarrassed at being caught out with an irrational fear: the point is not that no explanation can be offered but that one is required. If I had no reasons to tolerate the company of spiders but made no efforts to avoid them whatsoever, then it would make no sense to say that I feared them. On the other hand, my behaviour in avoiding spiders might be adequately explained by saying that I fear them and thus, if my fear is irrational, my behaviour is susceptible to rational criticism. If it is correct to equate moral attitudes with feelings of some sort, then it is clear that the feelings in question are more like emotions than tastes. Thus the claim that morality would not be possible unless we had feelings may be true and yet it does not show that reason has no role in morality, since we can and do have reasons for the ways we feel, reasons that can be examined and found to be good or bad. Nor does it show that reason cannot be used to criticise behaviour, since to the extent that we explain behaviour with reference to feelings, it is possible rationally to assess those feelings.

These considerations provide the basis for a positive account of morality when we consider that our concept of a rational being is that of a being that has feelings in this sophisticated sense. It is doubtful that we would, in any sense other than a metaphorical one, describe a computer as a 'rational being'. Rather, it in some ways resembles a rational being, in that it is capable of performing some of the cognitive functions (such as deduction) characteristic of such a being. Certainly it is not a rational agent, so it does not conform to what might be described as our fullest conception of a rational being. Similarly it can be argued that psychopaths are lacking in their understanding of the reality of other sentient beings. To be completely incapable of sympathy is to fall short of our full concept of a rational agent – at least if this incorporates the idea of a rational moral agent. The psychopath might conform to some more 'shallow' conception of rationality: in some sense he may be 'very rational'. But this is analogous to the sense in which a computer may be 'rational': it may be much better at deductive reasoning than the average human being but incapable of exhibiting any richer forms of reasoning.

Our concept of rationality (in the 'full' sense, which is surely what we mean when we talk about 'rational human beings') is a practical concept. It applies to the behaviour of persons, allowing us to evaluate it. To say a person is rational is not merely to say that certain processes are occurring 'in her head': it is to make a claim about the way she behaves, her attitude to those around her, her general disposition. So the claim that all voluntary behaviour is motivated by feelings, far from suggesting irrationalism, actually provides the basis for an account of morality which is not irrationalist. We can discuss the appropriateness of specific feelings/attitudes in specific contexts and we can ask whether or not there are any feelings that are essential characteristics of a rational agent. It should be the job of philosophy to examine such questions and to develop answers which can be helpful to us, not only in determining the conduct of our own lives as individuals but also in our thinking about the moral relationships we have with those around us, by considering what a morally decent society would look like. As we work out what manner of being rational moral agents are, we can ask questions about how such beings would treat each other, what sort of social arrangements they would develop and (perhaps more importantly) what types of arrangement could not possibly be acceptable to them. So the fact that morality is grounded in feelings both explains and (when properly understood) undermines the appeal of irrationalism. I will argue (Part Four) that a dispositional analysis of feelings (meaning, an understanding of feelings in terms of the characteristic way a person tends to react to the specific situations and problems she encounters) can provide the basis for a more convincing form of ethical intuitionism than the form considered already (Chapter 2). If the intuitionists had expressed their claims not in terms of certain moral propositions supposedly known by intuition but in terms of specific tendencies to react in certain ways then they would, in my view, have developed a more defensible approach to the issues of moral thinking and moral education.

To return to the analogy with epistemology (of Chapter 2) certain empirical data just strike me as evidence that whatever I am encountering is a real object, because I have the rational disposition to construe my experiences as experiences of a world which includes me as a small part of it; a world that pre-dates me and will certainly outlive me. This is not a 'mere preference' of mine. It is not an irrational predisposition. If I lacked this disposition I couldn't even get going as a rational being, so it is one of the things that defines my status as rational. To suggest that intuitions (meaning fundamental dispositions to believe, to think in certain ways) are necessarily irrational or non-rational is to make rationality itself impossible. While there are those who apparently sincerely view the denial of rationality as somehow intellectually 'liberating', this strikes me as about as sensible as attempting to 'liberate' me physically by removing my spinal cord. To lack any rational intuitions is to have lost the ability to distinguish sense from nonsense, to have become as intellectually and emotionally pliable as a model citizen of Orwell's Oceania (a spin doctor's ideal society). We need to hone our critical thinking skills, since they are our first and final defence against stupidity. We need philosophy. Instead of pronouncing practical reason dead, philosophers should turn their attention to investigating and promoting rational dispositions.

Some philosophers believe that the role of philosophy in practical discussion should be entirely critical: that we should spend our time (to adapt Locke's view about the relationship between philosophy and science) sweeping away some of the rubbish that stands in the way of progress, subjecting nonsense to analysis to expose it for what it is. I have a great deal of sympathy with this view, but the activity of sweeping away rubbish only makes sense on the assumption that there is something other than rubbish that might replace it. In Part Four I will attempt to say more about what this is in the context of health services management. It would be a mistake to think that, having disposed of the 'principles' of management science, it is either necessary or possible to make a 'positive' contribution by supplying some other set of principles, goals or guidelines in terms of which people can solve their problems. Rather, the 'rubbish' which philosophy sweeps away represents the barriers to sound intuitive thinking, for 'philosophy' here is construed primarily as a practice, rather than a body of propositional knowledge. We should not aim to supply a new set of 'answers' but instead we should strive to enable people to find good answers for themselves. The main reason for embracing the discipline of philosophy must be to develop and sustain the right sort of dispositions in ourselves and others. We must abandon the search for formulae to determine what is right or good, in exchange for investigating methods of intellectual and moral training that will equip individuals to think well and live well, despite all the barriers they are likely to encounter in the diverse situations they must face. We might call this view: philosophy as training in intellectual and moral self-defence.

Chapter 6

... And the rise of the 'ethicist'

This view of philosophy – as a form of training in intellectual and moral self-defence, a 'discipline' in the proper sense of the word – is by no means the dominant one amongst applied philosophers. Indeed, when I have presented it to gatherings of colleagues at other institutions, I have sometimes felt as if I were presenting Hume's arguments against the possibility of miracles to a group of evangelical faith healers. Typical reactions range from incredulity to open hostility and the main objection, sometimes stated in so many words, is that I am declaring applied philosophy 'impossible', thereby threatening to do us all out of a job.

On the face of it, this is a rather odd argument for philosophers to advance. Obviously, there is no credible theory of truth which implies that claims can only be true if their truth does not damage one's own employment prospects.[10] In any case, it is not at all clear why anything I have said implies the impossibility of applied philosophy: quite the reverse, in fact. It is the application of philosophical methods of thinking that provides our best defence against the stupidity and moral blindness that surrounds us. Acquire this discipline and steer a steady course between the twin ills of dogmatism, on one side ('I know what I think'), and on the other side that strain of intellectual 'flexibility' that makes one 'opinion fodder' – on whom the spin doctors and workplace ideologues may test their latest 're-educative initiatives' with impunity. In a complex world, what skill could be more necessary?

Why, then, do so many applied philosophers react in the way described? I think their reaction shows just how entrenched is a particular view of what it means to 'apply' theory to practice.

What gives offence is my claim that it is a 'mistake' to suppose that, in addition to exposing erroneous approaches such as 'quality management', philosophy can supply an alternative set of 'principles, goals or guidelines' for the ethical running of the health service. We live in an age obsessed with the production of regulatory frameworks, sets of guidelines, codes of practice and the like. On the basis of little or no evidence it is declared that spending massive amounts of money on producing such frameworks and then checking that everyone is following them (requiring the constant monitoring of people's behaviour) is the best way to improve practices in healthcare, education and elsewhere (Loughlin 2000a). So if clinicians are making bad decisions, instead of thinking carefully about creating environments and methods of training to enable them to make better decisions, it is assumed (with very little thought or argument) that what is needed is a 'single, authoritative source of advice' (Rawlins 1999, p. 1079) to health professionals and their managers. Hence the formation of such bodies as the National Institute for Clinical Excellence, whose wonderfully Orwellian abbreviation is of course 'NICE'. Although lip-service is sometimes paid to the idea of the 'reflective practitioner', in practice the use of individual judgement is increasingly discouraged. Thus the chairman of NICE warns that 'health professionals would be wise to record their reasons for non-compliance' with NICE guidelines in patients' medical records since such 'non-compliance' may precipitate an investigation by the CHI (Commission for Health Improvement, another title with a splendidly Stalinist ring to it).[11]

By fiat the social world is being divided into 'thinkers' and 'doers'. The doers do well if they follow the guidelines in their area, whatever they may be. 'I was only following procedure' becomes an automatic defence: even if the outcome was disastrous (and even if one feels that a properly trained practitioner should have known that in this case it would be disastrous) the practitioner was 'correct' to follow the guidelines – meaning, formally correct. The thinkers are supposed to devise the guidelines: otherwise what use are they? If their processes of deliberation do not produce any 'substantial conclusions', in the form of a set of 'dos' for the doers to 'apply', then it is taken as read that they are 'pure' intellectuals and have no contribution to make to 'real life'. This way a crude division between 'theory' and 'practice' becomes embedded in the structure of social and specifically professional life.

Against this background, my claim that what philosophy has to offer practitioners is not another set of guidelines but the skill of sustained critical thinking sounds dangerously unfashionable. Society may need critical thinkers but at the moment its behaviour suggests that what it wants is more formalistic rule followers. Perhaps people feel they have no time to think for themselves, that this is a 'luxury' they can seldom afford (rather than a necessity they cannot do without). Or perhaps they really do believe that it is not their business to think critically. Undoubtedly the social project described in Chapter 4, the attempt to reduce every aspect of life to a market transaction, reducing all moral relations and obligations to contractual relations and obligations, has much to do with this. If you 'know the rules' and keep them then you have done your duty, because we have almost lost contact with any more meaningful conception of duty that could define our nature as moral and social beings.

Because this is the social backdrop against which work in 'applied philosophy' takes place and because such work, like work in any other academic field, needs to attract funding if it is to continue, it is perhaps unsurprising that many applied philosophers have seen fit to demonstrate their 'usefulness' to the sources of funding by offering something they can recognise as 'substantial', rather than risk trying their patience by explaining to them why this is not necessarily desirable. Thus much of the work of applied philosophers in practice involves devising sets of principles or guidelines which purport to apply the already existing body of ethical theory to some morally problematic area of practice.

This has led to a proliferation of 'applied' disciplines of one sort or another. 'Medical ethics' and 'nursing ethics' are apparently branches of 'bioethics' (or 'biomedical ethics') but there are also 'healthcare ethics', 'business ethics', 'professional ethics' and 'organisational ethics'. All of them would seem to be branches of 'applied ethics', a term which is typically used interchangeably with 'applied philosophy'. There are academics who list as their 'specialist areas' two or three (or more) of these subjects, even though the distinctions between them, in terms of either methodology or content, are not always entirely clear. To become a specialist in one of these 'disciplines' it is necessary to add to one's knowledge of moral theories some empirical information about the specific professional context which generates the problems you aim to solve. Insofar as there is any distinction between the various forms of 'applied ethics' just listed, it is likely to be a function of this 'empirical' component to the discipline. So the 'applied' branch of philosophy becomes increasingly autonomous, and 'applied philosophy' can at times seem to be an altogether distinct practice from its 'pure' counterpart. (In a further development, the study of 'ethics' is sometimes distinguished from the study of 'philosophical ethics' and there are 'ethicists' who openly declare that they know nothing whatsoever about philosophy.[12])

In other words, my fellow applied philosophers frequently attempt the very thing which I have claimed philosophy should not do. The attempt to produce sets of ethical 'principles, goals or guidelines' to implement at the level of specific management decisions is that branch of 'professional ethics' called 'management ethics'. When such philosophers discuss the overall organisation of the health service their main role is to produce (often in collaboration with colleagues from other fields, most notably health economics) principles which will enable the government to ration resources more 'ethically'. So when I stand up in front of a group of applied ethicists, having helped myself to their coffee and biscuits and perhaps even expecting a meal later on, and tell them in all seriousness that ethical theory cannot be applied in this way, there is an understandable sense of outrage, even betrayal. The most common arguments advanced against me are as follows.

- I effectively collapse the distinction between 'pure' and 'applied' philosophy, leaving no room for applied philosophy.
- In doing so I am being rather 'negative' about what philosophy can and can't achieve. If it is possible to use philosophical methods to demonstrate that certain approaches are wrong, then why is it not possible to use the same methods to discover and implement the right approach? Why the asymmetry?

Both represent only a partial grasp of what I am actually claiming.

Pure and applied philosophy: an artificial distinction

If by 'applied philosophy' we mean to refer to a quasi-autonomous branch of philosophy, distinct from the 'pure' form of the subject from which it evolved, then this, it seems to me, is a bogus discipline. There is no such thing as either applied or pure philosophy in the sense implied. A theoretical approach does not become less theoretical by being 'applied' to something. Philosophical thinking always has content: there must always be a subject matter under discussion, if the discussion is to be about anything. Consider a discussion that might well be classified as 'pure' philosophy: for instance, certain fundamental questions of epistemology or questions of personal identity. We could answer questions about what can and cannot be known or about the nature of and identity conditions for human subjects by appeal to unquestioned dogmas or by thinking critically and analytically about them. Only if we take the latter option are we doing philosophy since, as we have seen, the discipline is characterised primarily by its methods, not its subject matter. An American 'televangelist' who screams at his audience that he 'knows' his soul is immortal, perhaps because God recently told him so, makes a contentious claim with implications for what sorts of thing can be known and for the nature of personal identity, but he is not thereby doing philosophy. Suppose Richard Dawkins runs onto the stage shouting 'fiddlesticks and flap-doodle!'[13] and a slanging match and punch-up ensue. Then we have a dispute about these contentious issues but it is not in any meaningful sense of the word a philosophical dispute.[14] (This is the serious point behind the old Monty Python sketch wherein the question of God's existence is settled by a wrestling match: 'God exists by two falls and a submission'.)

If we do take the latter option then we are applying philosophical methods to these important questions and so we may as well describe epistemology and the philosophy of mind as forms of 'applied philosophy'. Equally, we can apply philosophical methods to controversial moral questions and so long as we do so in an appropriately rigorous manner then we are doing philosophy, not some new or corrupted form of the subject: so we may as well call it 'pure philosophy'. On the other hand, we could answer such questions with reference to dogmatic assertions, in which case we are not doing 'applied philosophy' because we are not doing philosophy at all.

Therefore, the distinction has no proper application. We may as well abandon it. As noted above, the only distinction between the various forms of 'applied philosophy' seems to be in terms of the empirical matter which each named 'discipline' purports to address. The danger in the use of the term 'applied philosophy' is that the subject's identity becomes associated with the areas under discussion, rather than the distinctive style of thinking in terms of which the subject matter is understood, such that the word 'applied' philosophy becomes an excuse for 'bad' philosophy. Then any vacuous chit-chat about what 'should be done', however dogmatic and unreasoned, becomes 'applied ethics'.[15] We are already seeing the effects of this process, as forms of 'ethics' come into being which openly eschew any connection with philosophical methods, so we have people talking loosely about any subject with purported 'ethical' content and claiming 'expertise' in 'ethics' as a result.

This is potentially disastrous, because it means we are at risk of losing the most valuable feature of philosophical thinking – its ability to liberate us from sophistry and dogma – just where we should most expect to find it. Too many classes in 'applied ethics' consist of a simplistic characterisation of a problem, followed by a series of conjectures concerning what 'the consequentialist would say' about it, what 'the deontologist would say' about it, perhaps even what 'the Aristotelian would say' about it. It is as if there are clearly delineated bits of reality that constitute 'problems' and several clear formulae, represented by labels like 'deontology', which offer solutions to those problems. If there is any explanation offered for the selection of the particular problems (or 'dilemmas') for discussion it is likely to be that many people do in fact view these as the 'real' problems. For instance, many people see that, given scarce resources, there are real and perplexing moral questions concerning how to ration them, particularly when they are life-saving medical resources. Not so many people feel that the structure of society which determines the conditions of scarcity (and so the need for rationing), the social conditions under which so many people become so ill that they need to have their lives 'saved' and other 'deep' political concerns represent the really practical problems.

So it is usually considered more 'relevant' (to the unanalysed preconceptions of the audience) to discuss questions of the former type when doing applied philosophy. The fact that the theoretical characterisation of 'the problems' is selected with reference to (undoubtedly media-led) public opinion perhaps suggests one of the three controversial assumptions about the relationship between truth and belief, discussed above (Chapter 5). Something is taken to be a real problem just if it is perceived to be a problem by most people. That some form of relativism is implicit in many such discussions is further indicated by the fact that, once what each theory 'would say' has been identified, the choice of which theory to adopt is usually left to the student's personal preferences and little consideration is given to questions about which, if any, approximate to the truth.

What has been 'slipped by' the audience (be it a class of students or the readers of a text) is that initial characterisation and perhaps also the impression that the solutions offered represent all the 'credible' or 'realistic' possibilities. To call this process 'philosophy' is to do violence to the term, so perhaps it is a blessing that increasingly 'ethicists' reject the label 'philosophy'. It should not be necessary to argue (particularly when discussing social phenomena) that descriptions of 'the data' are laden with philosophical assumptions. Applying philosophical theory is not a matter of bringing a completed whole thing, a theory, to another thing called 'reality' whose nature is philosophically uncontroversial. As noted above (Chapter 1), to think at all is to conceptualise the data of experience in some way and there is no such thing as an atheoretical conceptualisation. So the attempt to characterise the practices one aims to evaluate is an attempt to organise the data of experience in accordance with some theory. At all levels the theory concerns reality and it is no less a theory the less general its concerns become. There is therefore no sharp distinction to be drawn between the development of the theory and its application: rather, the application of a theory is a further development of it and difficulties in applying a theory count as difficulties for the theory itself. Theories with implausible implications for practical problems are rendered implausible *as* theories. The claim that 'it works well in theory, but not in practice' represents a confusion, based on a false dichotomy between theory and practice: if the theory does not apply to anything then it does not work *in theory* either. What we should say instead is that what at first appeared to be a good theory turned out, after further consideration, not to be so good.

The 'asymmetry' objection: philosophers and 'ethicists' as apologists for the status quo

We can see what is wrong with the 'symmetrical' thinking behind the second objection noted above, by reconsidering the discussions of 'case studies' and 'professional codes' in Chapters 1 and 2 respectively. The question is not, can philosophical methods help individuals in practical situations find adequate answers to real moral questions? I have already argued that they can, by helping to liberate thinking from the influence of sophistry and dogma, and I shall say a good deal more about the practical application of philosophical thought in Part Four. (As we will see shortly, they can also help us to identify situations where there are no morally adequate solutions available and to work out how we should respond to such situations.) The issue at stake here is whether philosophical theory, or indeed any other theoretical approach, can produce principles or guidelines that can be directly applied to the resolution of real problems, to guarantee an 'ethical' outcome – in the way that one can follow the instructions of the TV repair manual and be reasonably confident that (if the authors of the manual 'know their stuff') the fault discovered will be corrected.

The reasons why this cannot be done are as follows:

- the contentious nature of the subject
- the need for subjective interpretation of any principle or code
- the irrational nature of the context which gives rise to the problems under discussion.

The first two reasons are implicit in what has gone before. I can, of course, just 'tell you' my position with respect to a particular moral controversy, but if I tell you my position 'as a moral philosopher' then I am probably playing a trick upon you. Ethics is a much more contentious subject than (for example) pharmacy. A philosopher can't just dispense answers to moral questions as if they were tried and trusted remedies, because the subject isn't like that. The substitution of the title 'ethicist' for 'moral philosopher' helps to disguise this fact, which is perhaps part of its appeal for those who adopt it: if you want something to alleviate the pain of your headache, seek the advice of a pharmacist; so if you want to alleviate the problems of social injustice, whose advice do you seek? Well obviously, an ethicist's.

Even if there were some uncontentious set of principles defining 'ethical practice' in health management or elsewhere, it would require interpretation before it could be applied. (Obviously an 'ethical code' which cannot be applied has no substantial implications.) But we have seen that the process of interpretation in any given context will depend in part upon awareness of context-specific information, such that no answer can be read off any set of principles or guidelines, however detailed, concerning situations of that general 'type'. Furthermore, the classification of a particular situation as an instance of a given type is a philosophically controversial exercise, requiring the employment of critical judgement. So even if I come to the conclusion that a particular moral theory is true, this cannot, in itself, tell me how to solve any real moral problems. The moral theories I accept can help to shape my views about moral life in very broad terms, but there is no straightforward relationship between acceptance of a given theory and how one reacts in any particular situation.

The third reason stated above requires a little more explanation. To claim it is possible to use philosophy (or indeed any rational method) 'to discover and implement the right approach' to the problems of the health service is to make an assumption about the context of health service decision making. It is to assume that one can, first of all, raise general questions about what health policy 'should be' and reasonably hope to be able to answer those questions rationally. Then, having developed a defensible conception of what an ethical health service would look like, one can start to think about how specific professional roles can function within that broader ethical structure, so determining what sorts of things people occupying those roles 'should do'.

While both types of inquiry may seem initially reasonable, I will argue that they are both doomed, given the irrational nature of the social context which gives rise to the problems they purport to solve. If these were the only conceivable ways to 'apply' philosophy then the project of 'applied philosophy' really would be impossible. In fact, the role of this form of 'ethics' (and it is a project which also very much involves those non-philosophical ethicists referred to above) is not to enlighten and support people trying to find morally adequate responses to problems generated by the professional roles they happen to occupy. Its real aim is to vindicate the roles themselves and the broader system of which they are a part. Again, it may seem natural to assume that these goals are one and the same or, at the very least, compatible. However, I will argue that appearances here are deceptive. To adopt the latter project – to attempt a formal vindication of certain social roles and the economic and social structures of which they are a part – is to assume the role of apologist for the status quo. To do this is to rule out of court consideration of the very questions which we must consider, whatever our particular profession, if we are to become responsible, reflective practitioners. Philosophy can only be of any real use to people if it enables them to understand the true nature and causes of the problems which confront them and to do this properly, it must require them to think honestly and critically about the roles they occupy and the forces and structures which shape those roles. Forms of 'applied ethics' which do not do this are at best practically useless and intellectually unsatisfactory. At worst, they may serve to confuse and mislead, so actually inhibiting moral and intellectual progress.

These arguments are set out below. While they have been welcomed enthusiastically by some practitioners, as already noted I have met mostly with opposition since I began to present these points, in papers and in informal discussion, to people working in the field of 'ethical theory'. Bioethicists have suggested that I contradict myself by apparently championing applied philosophy, only to declare it impossible. This is certainly what Dracopoulou (1998, p. 9) means to insinuate by contrasting my views about the need for philosophy with my criticisms of contemporary bioethics. (We will return to the substance of her criticisms in Part Four.) Management specialists complained that I was pronouncing managers 'incapable' of 'thinking ethically' (Wall 1998, p. 13). Despite considerable evidence to the contrary, Wall (1994, p. 318) declared that I was claiming only professional philosophers had the 'right' to talk about matters of 'right and wrong' and chastised me for the outrageous 'arrogance' of this view. In 'reply' he stated that managers have as much right as academics to discuss such matters (and as their 'mentor', he would apparently do much of the talking for them). Wall added that as 'practical' people, managers were 'well informed about the context of their work' but not about 'philosophical theories', which are not to the 'purposes' of people concerned with 'the more mundane processes of what is called "real life".' As an example of a properly 'practical' piece of writing he cited his own *Ethics and the Health Services Manager*, which he described as 'another text yet to be dismembered by Loughlin'[16] and which successfully avoids the construction of any coherent theoretical framework.

Given the preceding comments, we can perhaps see what is wrong with this dichotomy between having knowledge of a 'context' and having a theoretical framework. Any characterisation of a context embodies theoretical assumptions. In line with most management theorists, Wall treats his own assumptions as too obvious to merit honest articulation, let alone any defence. Because I actually attempt to defend what I say with arguments, I am described as 'arrogant'. In contrast, Wall makes a virtue of offering no arguments whatsoever for anything he says, expecting his readers to accept it simply because he describes himself as their 'mentor'. Despite myself, I cannot help but admire the man for constructing so wonderful a piece of sophistry.

Wall's reasoning is wonderful in another way: it provides an excellent illustration of the 'guidelines' approach to ethics, exposing (albeit unwittingly) the errors behind it. Once a crude opposition between 'theory' and 'practice' has been posited, theorising immediately becomes the activity of an elite minority and something which practitioners do not need. Viewed through such distorted conceptual lenses,[17] my claim that ethics requires critical thinking becomes the claim that most people cannot possibly think ethically. To anyone who has read thus far without the aid of Wall's conceptual glasses, it will be obvious that this in no way represents my view. I take the capacity to reason to be a fundamental feature of human thought, not the exclusive property of some professional group. As moral agents, we all have not the 'right' but the duty to think seriously about the moral status of our activities. You respect another person's status as a rational being by offering her arguments in support of the claims you make, since then she is able to assess your arguments herself and decide whether she can, in good conscience, accept them. You do not respect another person by telling her it is not her 'role' to think critically about the functions she performs, offering her a 'simple ethical framework' (Wall 1989, p. *ix*) in terms of which to live out her professional life, a framework which you do not bother to defend because you regard her as a person with 'vague and half-digested ideas' (Wall 1994, p. 318) who could not understand complex reasoning anyway. Clearly it is not my position that is arrogant and patronising. Unlike Wall, I do not think of my audience as the 'intellectually incompetent' (op cit). My goal is the promotion of critical thinking as widely as possible, not its restriction to a narrow group of academics, so Wall (misled by his own assumptions) 'replies' to a position that is quite the reverse of my own.[18]

Bioethics and the irrationality of the social world

I have argued elsewhere (Loughlin 1995a, p. 43) that applied philosophers must consider the question 'who is my audience?'

if they are to clarify the aims of their activity and to understand their own presuppositions when they write articles and engage in debate. I suggested three possible answers which can be summarised as follows:

1 other academics
2 politicians and the powerful
3 a 'wider audience', by which I meant any rational human able to understand the arguments put forward and willing to take them seriously.

The first answer would suggest that one's primary aim in doing applied philosophy is to gain academic prestige and to enjoy whatever pleasures arise from convincing one's academic peers by valid arguments that one is right about something. Giving the second answer would suggest that one hopes to use philosophy to influence the decisions of policy makers and so to bring about some desirable consequences. The third answer implies the aim of 'enabling people to question traditional ways of conceptualising problems' so as 'to raise the general level of thought and discussion in society' (op cit).

It is worth revisiting this question since the statements of some of bioethics' most distinguished proponents[19] suggest that they would give the wrong answer. That is, they would answer that, as far as so-called 'pure' philosophy is concerned, 1 is the correct answer but when philosophy is being applied to the 'real world' then 2 is the right answer – although obviously one expects (or hopes) that one's work will be studied by one's colleagues in each case. From what has gone before it should be obvious that I would take 3 to be the right answer in each case (and I would reject the pure/applied distinction anyway).

As we have seen, 1 to 3 are not the only possible answers. Much of the work in bioethics is quite explicitly aimed at particular professional groups, be they doctors, nurses or (more recently) managers, and seeks to give advice to a limited readership on how to develop adequate moral responses to problems peculiar to that readership. Its prescriptions are directed neither at academics nor policy makers, nor are they valid for human beings as such, but rather they are valid for persons who occupy specific social roles. The attempt to construct a subject called

'the ethics of health services management' (Dracopoulou 1998)
is a project of this sort.

It seems obvious that, for any given problem under consideration, one possible conclusion of an inquiry of this sort will be
that there are no morally adequate solutions. An intellectually
honest doctor, nurse or manager must surely recognise that
certain problems she encounters within her social role are
determined by features of that role which are simply, from her
point of view, given and as a result the solutions typically
adopted are just plain arbitrary, no better or worse than any of
the available alternatives because none of them represents a
truly acceptable option. Nor is it clear, even, that there must be
some meaningful way to determine which of the options available is the 'lesser' of evils, since there is no reason to assume
that the world is so designed as to make rational answers to
every moral question possible.

I suspect, however, that a bioethicist who comes up with that
sort of answer too often will be deemed to have failed: to succeed
in bioethics is to provide principles or 'decision making tools'
that are 'practical', which means that they work within the
context given, rather than complaining that the scope for
rational thought is too limited by that context for its application
to be meaningful. Implicit is the assumption that the context
does not create problems that resist rational solution. But there
is no reason why this should not be so. There is no reason why
'What is the right (or best) thing for a person in role X to do
in circumstances ABC?' will necessarily have a determinate
answer. Indeed, given the largely arbitrary, non-rational processes which shape professional roles, it is highly unlikely
that this will always, or even very often, be the case.

The very existence of bioethics assumes that this is, at least,
often the case. The assumption is dogmatic and, as I will
argue, ideological. It reflects the view that social reality is
inherently rational, that its nature is determined by rational
processes. While it might seem desirable that this should be
so, we do not make it so by assuming that it is already. As I
have argued, it clearly is not so in contemporary society, not
even to the extent that the nature of that reality is determined
by public debate. For that debate is conducted in largely
irrationalist terms.

In its attempt to provide 'realistic' solutions to the problems of practice, (meaning, ones that are adequate given the nature of the world as it is) bioethics masks the arbitrary, irrational nature of much of social reality. It may often be that when faced with such problems, the best that philosophy can do is give sense to individuals' feelings of frustration, to articulate the sense that no matter what you do there is no satisfactory answer and to confirm that far from being 'negative' and 'unhelpful', such feelings represent the most rational, objective and human response: indeed, they are a prerequisite for understanding the truth about one's predicament and finding ways to cope with it. In this way philosophy can offer support to individuals placed in impossible situations by enabling them to understand the causes of their difficulties. It may well be that if I cannot find the right answer or if none of the options available seem acceptable, this is not because I am being unreasonable but because my world is unreasonable and I am sufficiently sane to have noticed. Such a realisation is the very beginning of critical thought. Life often seems senseless because it often is senseless: when the conditions of life are determined largely by irrational processes it is no surprise that rational life feels so much of the time like an ongoing struggle against stupidity. This is what it is.

To think in this way is to think beyond one's specific roles, to make those roles, and the social structure which gives rise to them, the object of moral and intellectual criticism. There is still much to be said about how, having assumed such a broader perspective, one then reintegrates this perspective with one's specific position within the structure, but this is the necessary first stage in thinking philosophically. (To return to the dominant analogy of Chapter 1, this is to begin to draw the map.) One cannot meaningfully claim to be thinking autonomously until one has made this first step. And one can only function as a moral agent when one has begun to think autonomously. We cannot treat 'ethics' as construction of moral codes for members of specific professional groups, the implication being that when such codes are developed and followed people will be behaving 'rationally' and 'ethically'. This idea could only make sense if the rational significance of the relevant professional roles were clear; if, instead of being shaped by a variety of possibly conflicting historical forces, these roles were created for a clearly understood moral purpose, having a place within some rational social design. Otherwise, the codes are more likely to function as a substitute for critical, rational thinking.

It makes sense, then, that bioethicists are interested in more 'holistic' questions, concerning the overall design of healthcare systems and how it might be made more rational. This involves discussing general issues of health service policy, such as how roles should be allocated to different professional groups within healthcare and how scarce resources should be rationed. If only we could come up with an overall picture of how an ethical service would operate, we could work out how resource allocation decisions at the microeconomic level would fit in and what role each specific group would play in implementing those decisions.

The question is, what sort of debate is being envisaged here? Clearly, I could indulge any number of fantasies about how an ideal service might function. I could imagine a context in which all needs could be met, where the senseless and the unspeakable were never unavoidable – where, for instance, it was never 'necessary' for an old man to die horribly and alone waiting for a service which (to steal some lovely prose from the IHSM) 'this society' is no longer 'willing to afford'. Further, I could imagine a world in which he never suffered from the grotesque condition which killed him, because his employers were not so cruel and miserly as to make him work such long hours up to his chest in filthy polluted water, with such cheap inadequate protective equipment. Or I could more modestly imagine a world in which he did not have to be alone at the end, because his local authority could at least afford someone clinically unqualified to visit him more often, perhaps if the home help service had not been decimated by recent 'quality reforms'.

But such utopian dreaming is not the stuff of serious bioethical debate. The bioethicist is empirically minded: he takes the real world as his starting point. This is important. To be 'realistic' in the context of a debate about 'bioethics' means to attempt to show how, given the world as it is, we can find 'ethical' solutions to the problems of health services organisation and policy. For the debate to have any substance, the current state of society, and of the health service, must be taken as a 'given' and not subjected to moral questioning. If we ask why salaried people are so greedy, so short-sighted and so wilfully blind to the suffering of the worst off in society that they think savings on income tax make the gradual destruction of the public services well worth it, then we are, quite simply, not doing 'bioethics'. Unlike real philosophy, where one must follow a line of questioning through to its logical conclusion, wherever it goes, in this area it is essential to learn to come to a halt at certain points which mark out the limits of one's academic remit.

This brand of 'realism' may seem to some to be the great strength of bioethics, but I will argue that this is not so much a realistic stance as it is an uncritical one. The result is a subject which bears certain similarities to philosophy, adopting some of its terminology and often (certainly amongst philosophically trained bioethicists) its characteristic style of argument, but which lacks its key virtue in questioning fundamental presuppositions. The relationship between bioethics and philosophy is like that between a Victorian folly and a real castle: the copy fails to fulfil the central function of the original. It no more provides a defence against dogma than most of the silly monuments to their supposed cultural superiority could have provided the Victorians with security in the face of a real assault. By offering solutions to practical problems via rational methods, ethicists confirm that 'rational' and 'ethical' solutions are possible within the present political environment: it is not that the environment must change radically if reason is to survive at all, but rather rational debate can flourish provided it accepts certain arbitrary limits placed upon it. By agreeing to work within the confines of 'realistic' assumptions, such theorists may find that their work functions to underwrite the very conceptions of reality and practice which must change if social rationality is even to be possible.

The rationing debate

The academic agenda of bioethics is determined by the agenda of the powers that be. This is why the question of how to ration scarce resources is so important and so frequently discussed within the subject. While the Western powers can find any amount of money to fund bombardments of countries whose leaders have fallen out of favour, as far as health resources are concerned economic scarcity is a 'fact of life', so governments search for rationales to deny access to those services to some groups within the population. As noted in Chapter 4, it is currently unfashionable to give a Marxist analysis of any social phenomenon. Even so, it is perhaps worth pointing out that what is in origin an economic problem for governments has (as a Marxist might expect) given rise to a flurry of intellectual activity in the field of moral philosophy, as academics construct theories of justice in resource allocation to prove that fair methods do in fact exist to ration essential health resources as (it just so happens) the economy requires.

The process is often described in rather more sanitised terms as 'priority setting', a title which has the advantage of making the whole procedure sound a little less grim and a little more scientific than in fact it is. Frequently the relative claims of different groups to a share of the service's limited resources are assessed in terms of their rights, needs or capacity to benefit and principles or purpose-built theoretical devices (such as the economists' QALY) are proposed as solutions to the problem of how to ration ethically. The aim is to enable the ethical policy maker (notably, often identified with 'we', the moral community – an identification typically treated as unproblematic) to discriminate systematically and in the least offensive way possible, whether it is the elderly, those who have 'irresponsible lifestyles', those whose treatments are expensive or some other, less easily identified but nonetheless real group of persons who are singled out for inconvenience, suffering and even death. Thus it is taken as read that the goal of the debate is to produce recommendations to improve practice: the point is (to parody Marx) not simply to *explain* the problems of the health service but to *change* the service for the better.

What is more, the changes recommended must be 'realistic', meaning that they must be achievable within the economic constraints upon the service which frame the debate. So contributors do not view it as morally outrageous that some people who could in principle be relieved will instead suffer and die.

The pain, terror and despair of the 'de-prioritised' are of course 'regrettable' but it is not the moral problem which contributors to the debate set out to address. The problem, rather, is the unsystematic way in which such pain, terror and despair are currently distributed. It is the lack of any theoretical rationale for this distribution which apparently gives offence. So-called 'postcode prescribing' was viewed with genuine moral outrage by most commentators because it seems so evidently 'arbitrary': people in Blackpool may be treated if they have condition X but not condition Y, while people in Teesside may be treated for condition Y but suffer unaided with condition X. If everyone, across the board, were treated for condition X and no-one were treated for condition Y this would look more formally consistent, more 'rational': although it is by no means clear why people in Blackpool suffering with condition Y should now feel satisfied that their pain and despair, though just as real, are somehow less 'arbitrary' than before, because even if they were living in Teesside they would still be suffering. Much less is it clear why people living in Teesside suffering with condition Y should rejoice at the overall formal consistency of the 'improved' system.[20]

Much of the theoretical debate concerns what it means for the service to be better: does this mean more 'fair' according to some specific conception of justice (the Rawlsian conception[21] being currently the most fashionable)? Or does the service's being better amount to its producing more benefits (raising obvious questions about what we mean by, and how we are to measure, benefit)? Even theorists who purport, however implausibly, to be engaged in 'value-neutral analysis' when discussing healthcare policy invariably comment on what it is right, best or most rational to do, given the assumption of certain goals whose nature and legitimacy are taken as uncontroversial (Williams 1995, pp. 221–2). For an exposure of the spurious nature of economists' claims to be 'value-neutral' see Seedhouse (1995) and Loughlin (1998a). If such theorists will not admit to being 'evaluative' they can substitute the word 'practical' since for our present purposes they mean the same thing: an evaluative discourse is one that aims to affect practice via the process of argument. It seems obvious that the arguments in question should be rational ones, since it is not clear how we can expect people to take what we say seriously unless we can provide them with good reasons to do so, and the attempt to influence practice by presenting good reasons for one's conclusions is an attempt to construct rational arguments.

Despite the undoubtedly honourable intentions of many of its contributors, it strikes me that this debate is, in an important sense, misguided. I will argue that the attempt to provide an account of the decision making processes which form general health service policy that is at once 'realistic' (taking the service as it is as its starting point) and 'pragmatic' (aiming to affect its nature via rational moral argument) fails, given the real nature of the context in which the decisions under discussion take place. The very idea that such an account might be possible derives from an assumption (to be spelled out in detail in what follows) which is both ideological in character and patently false. Indeed, it is only because the assumption in question is embedded firmly in the ideology dominant in our culture that it normally escapes critical attention, such that its influence and evident falsity remain unrecognised. Theorists who write in this area have to face the possibility not only that their work cannot do any positive good, but also that it may be positively harmful, in that it serves to endorse some of the central myths of contemporary society and so, by its very existence, threatens to distort that which it purports to analyse. If I am right, then we have to think very carefully about how we are to discuss the problems of the health service, in order to say anything that is at once true and worth saying. This task may be far more difficult than some theorists are prepared to admit.

In defence of negativity

This conclusion will strike many readers as very 'negative' and some will view this as a problem for my argument (rather than viewing the argument as presenting a problem for the assumptions it criticises). There is a common tendency in any 'practical' discussion to view an analysis as having failed (or at least as being somehow incomplete) if it has 'failed to come up with' any positive conclusions. Readers who react in this way should think very carefully about what it means to criticise an argument for having negative conclusions. Do they think that a 'negative' conclusion is less likely to be true than a 'positive' one? Is it that the truth doesn't matter, that 'being positive' is all that matters?

Such a response is ideological and deeply reactionary. We all know the sort of regime which insists that all news must be good news. The view that all arguments must be 'positive' is a peculiar academic variant on this theme. It has its basis in a consumerist view of the social world which now seems to permeate our thinking on almost every issue. On this view, the purpose of a piece of writing cannot be naively to state the truth, in an attempt to communicate with other rational beings who have the desire to understand their world. Rather, what one says, to be worth saying at all, must be 'useful'. What is more, the conception of 'usefulness' at work here (unlike conceptions of usefulness employed in more credible forms of philosophical pragmatism) implies that what one says must be of use to some group whose role is defined in terms of the existing social order, such as the role of the policy maker or manager. Only then can one's argument have a 'market' and only then can one be justified in stating it in the first place. So a critique of the social order which gives rise to these roles, which defines their nature and goals, can be dismissed out of hand: not because it is wrong but because there is no readily identifiable 'target group' to 'buy' its conclusions.

Thus it becomes impossible to criticise the prevailing social and economic order or to identify it as the main obstacle in the way of human beings searching for humane solutions to the problems they encounter. Since the target audience is identified in terms of their specific social functions, it becomes impossible to get people to think 'beyond their roles' in the way that I have argued they must if they are to think ethically at all. All arguments are set the task of proving how, given the established order, real and meaningful solutions to pressing moral problems can be found. The statement 'the system works' acquires by default the status of a logical truth, since what it is for any proposed solution to 'work' has to be explained with reference to the system as it is: either an argument does or does not make the attempt to show that morally adequate solutions can be found by working within the limits on human action defined by the system as it is. If it does not, then it can for that very reason be dismissed as not 'practical'. Radical criticisms of the dominant system and its ideology are often rejected, it is claimed, because they are not practical. The truth is quite the reverse: they are not considered practical *because* they are incompatible with that system and its ideology. The ideological framework rules out consideration of any alternative to itself and so appears to be no more than 'common sense' to those working within it.[22]

We have already seen this mentality at work in the apparently *ad hoc* linguistic legislation and verbal tinkering that characterises contemporary management theory (Part Two), much of which is a liturgy of positive thinking (imploring us to 'focus positive', to speak not of 'weaknesses' or 'failings' but of 'areas for improvement', to use words which 'empower action', to be 'obsessed' not with the world as it is and the horrors it contains but with our inspirational 'vision' of how it might be . . .). The desire to be positive also explains the attractiveness of the term 'priority setting' in contrast to 'rationing'. Any rational creature with finite means sets priorities: talking in this way enables us to focus on that which is achieved, rather than dwelling on failures. Our intellectual starting point becomes not a highly developed complex service already providing many forms of care but rather, we begin by thinking of a blank sheet, a scenario in which nothing is provided. This mental shift serves the same psychological purpose as the phrase 'today is the first day of the rest of your life'. We are invited to imagine ourselves starting as if from nothing, at the dawn of a new day, with everything still to do. Then, instead of deciding which services have to be cut, we think about which to provide. Against this benchmark any provision at all becomes an achievement. The implicit comparison with a single, rational creature deciding which goals to set itself helps us to forget that the 'de-prioritised' services are not simply goals which we (the 'rational community') have – temporarily or permanently – decided prudently to give up but that they represent depriving some individuals of the means of a bearable existence and sometimes of life itself. As I shall argue, it also encourages us to delude ourselves about our powers: specifically, about the locus of decision making in our own societies.

Even authors who talk a great deal of sense about this subject seem determined to be 'positive' about the topic and so to avoid expressions such as 'rationing'. Despite using the word in the title of his paper, Klein (1993, p. 96) suggests that the word 'rationing' is too 'emotional'. The prevailing idea, which comes across most strongly in the works of authors such as Williams (1995), is that if we get upset about the fact that people have to suffer and die, this somehow must cloud our judgement. It is somehow bad taste to make a fuss about such things which are, after all, 'necessary'. If we despair of finding an adequate solution (meaning, please note, a 'non-arbitrary' way to *distribute* such suffering) this only indicates our lack of moral and/or intellectual stamina – rather than, for instance, clear-sightedness and intellectual honesty. There has to be a solution: that is 'pure common sense'.

There is very little in this world that is absolutely necessary: most of the things we call 'necessary' are only necessary given certain conditions. It is both astonishing and revealing that many theorists writing about health seem to be of the opinion that it is not their business to examine critically the conditions which necessitate the problems they discuss. Whether they realise it or not, such theorists assume the role of apologists for, and servants to, the status quo. Their 'practical' work involves helping the whole machine tick over effectively or, failing that, explaining that the reason why it does not tick over right now is because no-one has yet thought of the theory which will fix it: there is simply no question that the machine may have a structural fault, that it is beyond fixing – however many broken bodies it churns out.

My arguments aim to be useful not to people who think that someone in their position 'should know' certain stock solutions to certain types of ethical problem, but to any human being who has the wisdom to feel humbled in the face of an increasingly baffling and unstable social world, who thinks: where do I start? – who refuses to take it for granted that he has all the right questions, let alone the right answers. Such a person has the right intellectual instincts to benefit from the discipline of philosophy.

To recap: good philosophy analyses the fundamental assumptions which underlie a discourse and philosophy can take any serious human discourse as the object of its study – be it religious discourse, scientific discourse or the language of specific practical moral arguments. We have seen that the assumptions studied are often treated as too obvious to be worthy of serious critical attention by those engaged in the discourse and yet it is possible to examine them for coherence and plausibility and, indeed, to discover that they do not stand up well to scrutiny: they may turn out to be highly controversial or even palpably false.

Further, we have seen that this way of thinking will be attractive to any rational being with the desire to understand his or her own situation and the wider context of which it is a part. It enables us to think not only within the confines of the roles and positions we happen to occupy but also to treat those roles and the structure in which they have their being as the object of our study. By thinking in this way we may find that we are able to gain a greater insight into the real nature of our problems and perhaps even to discover that their solution, also, lies beyond the limits of the roles we presently perform. This may be an uncomfortable realisation. It may be a huge task to work out how one responds to such a realisation. Nonetheless, the activity which gives rise to it is a prerequisite for reflective human thought and one cannot develop a meaningful response to one's own condition until one has taken the trouble to reflect seriously on what, precisely, one's condition is.

Pragmatism, realism and the easy solution

The intellectual character of the rationing debate is shaped and limited by certain assumptions of market economics, the key one being the central economic assumption of 'scarcity'. The moral case for an economic solution to the problems of rationing is stated most effectively by Alan Williams, who regards the debate as an attempt to discover how practice:

> 'ought to be conducted, in the face of scarcity, if our objective is to maximize the benefits of healthcare.'
> (Williams 1995, p. 221)

Because health resources are scarce, it would be wrong to waste them. An inefficient use of resources in one area leads inevitably to others being deprived of services they need: hence the moral imperative to find the most efficient (meaning 'cost-effective') organisation of services (Williams 1992). This view makes sense of the assumption of many management theorists that the role of health services management should be to introduce 'economic rationality' to the health service, incorporating the ethos of the market into the day-to-day running of the health service.

Any attempt to reason seriously about what 'efficiency' means in this context will encounter a variety of deep conceptual problems. To do the job properly it would be necessary to develop a theory that allowed us to measure the value of the many diverse benefits of different healthcare activities, in sufficiently precise terms to be able to feed them into a cost–benefit calculation. Apart from the apparently insurmountable epistemological problems in knowing how specific interventions affect the lives of diverse patients and the total absence of any adequate theory of value or account of the nature of benefit that could make quantification meaningful, the task seems to be rendered logically impossible since all too often we are dealing with incommensurable values. Even management theorists occasionally admit this:

> 'How can anyone choose between more staff for the special care baby unit and additional domicilary care for the elderly mentally confused; they have nothing in common but are equally deserving.' (Wall 1989, p. 43)

In addition to the problems in identifying and measuring benefits, there are deep problems involved in identifying and measuring costs, especially once we accept that not all costs are financial. As we have seen (Chapter 5), it is not clear how one measures the psychological and material damage suffered by persons (and their families) deprived of employment as a result of 'labour-saving' management innovations. What value (or rather disvalue) ought we to place upon the stress and sense of 'alienation' suffered by carers forced to work to 'productivity' targets which seem to them not only irrelevant to the nature of their work but blind to its true value (Darbyshire 1993)? The very attempt to put a figure on such costs would seem to falsify their nature: like so many features of human life, to treat them as something which one can quantify is to fail to understand them.

One standard theoretical response to such difficulties (with a long pedigree in economic theory) is to ignore them. Features of the context which cannot be quantified can, it is assumed, be left out of the calculation, but a meaningful calculation can still be performed. Here, theory seems to be dictating the nature of reality in a disturbing sense, since we effectively treat as unreal any features of the world which cannot be incorporated into our cost–benefit analysis. It makes little sense to say that I have a 'good' explanation of a series of events because I ignore all the evidence which my explanation cannot account for; just so, it seems entirely *ad hoc* to claim that we can have an adequate theory of decision making based on a device for measuring value, because we systematically ignore all the features of the world to which our device is insensitive. The only possible justification for giving such a response is the assumption that there must be some adequate way of making these decisions and, given the nature of social reality, appeal to such devices represents the only practical way of doing this. The 'best answer available to us' must, it is assumed, be 'adequate' and must effectively be treated as the 'right' answer, since the idea that neither the right, nor even the adequate, answers are available to us, given the system as it is, must be ruled out in advance.

The problem is only exacerbated if we insist that there are other essential requirements on an ethical organisation, in addition to efficiency. It may well be that there is more to the rationing debate than the question of how to maximise benefits, since even the maximally beneficial distribution (if one had some way of determining what this might be) could be objected to on the grounds that it was unjust (Chadwick 1993, p. 85). This generates further potentially intractable problems. We then have to decide not only who can benefit most from some specific type of treatment (taking all possible alternative benefits and costs into account) but also who has the most 'right' to it where, it seems, there is more to having the right to a given benefit than having the capacity to be benefited or harmed by the result of the decision: more, even, than being the person who would benefit more from the treatment in question than anybody else.

As economists never tire of pointing out, one solution not available is to deny the existence of scarcity or to complain that if we only spent more money on health the problem would go away. This is hard to deny, although more attention should be given to the question of precisely why this is the case. It seems essential to the nature of contemporary society that it generates more sickness than it can cure. Short of a radical change in the nature of society, which would abolish the problem and make all proposed solutions superfluous, there will always be some people with needs that could, in principle, be met but which will not be met in practice because there are many more legitimate claims on the service than it can satisfy.

This characterisation of the problem suggests one, rather swift, solution which for convenience I shall refer to as 'the easy solution'. One could argue that, since 'ought' implies 'can', and since a legitimate claim is one that ought to be met, not all of the claims on the service can really be legitimate since they cannot all be met. Those claims which the service cannot meet are not, therefore, legitimate claims.

To borrow a phrase from Bertrand Russell, this solution has all the advantages of theft over honest toil. How can a claim, which would otherwise be judged legitimate, become illegitimate as a result of factors which have nothing to do with the needs of the (potential) patient? Either those needs provide the basis for a legitimate claim or they do not. If they do not then there is no legitimate claim on the service, even if the resources are available. If they do (and the whole rationing debate is predicated on the reality that there are many such claims which cannot be met) then how can their legitimacy be wiped away by extraneous economic factors? If my lifestyle is such that I cannot pay all my debts, does it follow that they cannot really be my debts after all? Might we not conclude that I should change my lifestyle? Verbal games cannot disguise the fact that real people, with real needs, are being made to suffer and if this turns out to be an inevitable consequence of the nature of the society in which they live, then why not conclude that there is something fundamentally wrong with that society?

The problem with a society, in contrast to at least some human individuals (the ones, significantly, that we view as possessing rational self-control), is that it is not easy to get it to 'change its ways': the very idea that a complex society can simply decide, on the basis of a rational argument, to make fundamental changes to its internal organisation is based on an unrealistic view of the processes of social change. This point is often recognised but its implications for the nature of rational debate about society, and the limitations it places on such debate, often go unrecognised. The difficulties in using reason to effect change in the structure of society give rise to difficulties for the project of rationally effecting change in any substantial sector of the whole structure. To abstract that sector from the structure which gives it its being, to treat it in isolation, ignores the important relationships it has with the rest of the structure and so one is able to have a 'pragmatic' discussion, presenting proposals for practical change, at the expense of realism. (Therefore one's pragmatism is deluded.) The more realistic one becomes, the more one recognises the relationships with wider features of the whole which determine the nature of the sector under discussion, the more implausible it becomes to assume that one can change the nature of this reality by proving that it could, in so many ways, be much better. However impeccable the proof, there is no relationship between the impeccability of an argument and its causal efficacy in facilitating social change.

We find this tension between pragmatism and realism hard to accept; the vast majority of academic arguments ignore it altogether. This may be partially due to frustration: we find it hard to reconcile the idea that some feature of our own society could and should be better with the assertion that we are in no position to make it any better. However, the correct way to deal with frustration cannot be to deny the nature of the reality which frustrates one's hopes or ideals. It is interesting that we do not have any such problem when thinking about societies other than our own. We are happy to entertain the idea that many societies in history (doubtless ones 'less developed' than ours) may have been afflicted by problems which they simply could not solve, because the conditions were not right for an adequate solution to be found and implemented. There is a Hegelian[23] tendency to see one's own society as the end-product of the whole process of evolution and so to assume either that it cannot get any better or that, if it can, the means to make it better are readily available to its inhabitants, if they'll just give it some thought.

I'll return to this assumption shortly. For the moment I want to return to the easy solution. It is obvious that it will not do but it is worth thinking for a moment about why it will not do. It provides us with no systematic way of making the relevant decisions about who must suffer and/or die. It simply tells us that whichever decisions we make, we can retrospectively judge them to have been right, since those we chose to deprive of care had no legitimate claim in the first place, by virtue of the very fact that they were not selected. It is the sort of argument which old-fashioned philosophy books would call an 'apology', only it is not an apology for any specific position or decision but rather for any position on this issue which those making the decisions might care to take up. If they decide to discriminate against the elderly, then they can argue that they are right to do so. If they decide to discriminate against the young, then again they are right. The argument does not so much guide as rubber-stamp decisions. It is absurd to describe any argument as providing a 'defence' of a particular position or decision if it equally counts as a defence of the contrary position or decision. An argument which is compatible with both X and −X does not establish either. An argument which justifies anything you like justifies nothing in particular.

In contrast, then, a good argument would be one which determines a particular decision by giving it an adequate theoretical basis. That is to say, one should be able to deduce determinate answers to questions about how one ought to allocate health resources; ones that could be directly applied to practice. One should be able to say that certain decisions are (or would be) the right ones, and others would be wrong, and to provide a justification for that claim in terms of the theory of ethical decision making offered. Otherwise, what precisely is the theoretical debate about? If the work of theorists does not provide a clear method for criticising some decisions and for advocating others, then it does not really affect practice, except by creating the appearance that decisions made have a grounding in theory.

Bearing this in mind, it is worth looking at a couple of arguments which may be attractive to some practitioners precisely because they create the appearance that there is an adequate theoretical basis for decisions in practice. They invite people to go through a process of deliberation before making decisions, but the process does not determine any particular decision, nor does it in fact determine any specific attitude towards life in general which could then affect decisions. Having contemplated the theoretical arguments, decision makers are still obliged to choose on the basis of their own subjective reactions, just as they would have done had they never encountered the theory. What it offers them is a bogus sense of reassurance that they have some ethical 'grounding' which they didn't have before. This can then be used as a weapon in argument whenever their decisions are questioned. So these arguments are essentially similar to the easy solution but because they are expressed in more complex terms their logical status is not as readily apparent. The Russellian retort does not acknowledge that some types of theft can be hard work. If the easy solution is analogous to snatching a wallet and running at top speed, the solutions I want to consider now are akin to corporate fraud.

Illusory solutions: Wall's 'principles'

The first solution I want to look at concerns specifically the project of constructing an 'ethic for health services management' and can be found in Andrew Wall's book *Ethics and the Health Services Manager*. This solution is interesting because Wall apparently accepts the points I have been making about the incommensurability of values and the limits on rational thought in the context of the modern health service. He states:

> '*Obviously, choosing ways to spend [health] resources is not a rational process. It is largely influenced by assumptions and powerful groups, all as potent as they are non-rational.*' (Wall 1989, p. 101)

Wall has since explicitly rejected the idea that rationality has anything to do with management (Wall 1994). It would surely follow from this that no statement about how managers 'ought' to conduct themselves could be capable of justification since, as I argued above, the attempt to give good reasons for one's conclusions is the attempt to construct rational arguments. If the latter is impossible in the context of health service management, then so is the former. In which case, it follows that no-one can have any reason to take seriously anything Wall or anyone else has to say on the subject of what managers 'ought to do'. The discipline 'the ethics of health services management' is therefore impossible.

Undeterred, Wall (as noted in Part One) purports to offer 'practical guidance' to managers about how to conduct themselves 'ethically', by taking certain 'everyday dilemmas' and examining them 'within a simple ethical framework' (Wall 1989, from the Preface). He posits several 'principles', asserting that patients have certain 'rights' including:

- 'that their individuality be respected'
- 'that those looking after them should exert their best skills on the patient's behalf'

and

- 'that no unreasonable harm should come to them' (Wall 1989, p. 11).

At several points, Wall accepts that such statements do not have a very clear and direct application to practice. For instance, he admits that the definition of what is 'reasonable' is 'crucial' but instead of going on to provide the crucial definition, he gives an instance of expenditure which, in his view, is not reasonable (ibid, p. 15).

Naturally, Wall refuses to give a philosophical justification for his 'principles', stating that 'matters of moral philosophy' are not his concern (ibid, p. 2). The attempt to discuss ethics without getting involved in questions of moral philosophy is the intellectual equivalent of discussing how to build and maintain nuclear power stations, without getting bogged down in abstract discussion of theoretical physics. What exactly is accomplished? Does one have an 'ethical grounding' for one's decisions simply on the basis of having read a book with the word 'ethics' in the title? Little consideration, if any, seems to be given to the question of what it might mean to speak of an 'ethic for managers' and what conditions there are on the adequacy of any such 'ethic'. Is it meaningful to purport to 'guide' people when one accepts that no arguments can be offered to explain why anyone should follow one's 'guidance'? Is there a difference between 'ethical guidance' and 'a set of unsupported (and unsupportable) assertions'? Of course, Wall does not need to offer any defence of his 'principles' since they are phrased in such general terms that no-one in their right mind could disagree with them. (How many people think that unreasonable harm should befall patients or that those looking after them should not use their 'best skills' in doing so?) Wall avoids giving detailed explanations of how these principles apply to practice, expecting instead that his readers will use their judgement when applying them. In other words, the gap between the principles and practice is to be bridged by the subjective decisions of particular managers and two managers, supposedly using the same principles, could come to different decisions.

By now the similarities with the easy solution should be apparent. Anyone can issue a series of prescriptions or assert the existence of certain 'ethical principles' without argument. Such assertions could only have any merit if they were part of a theoretically adequate approach to solving moral problems. An adequate approach must either give a determinate answer to a specific question or it must provide a method which could generate some determinate answer in some specific situation. If my theory is so vague that it can be used to justify anything then it adds nothing to the debate, except the feeling that problems have been solved when clearly they haven't. Wall offers managers the chance to come to any decision they like and to say that it is justified in terms of ethical principles, should they feel the need to do so. The same feature which accounts for the work's popularity also guarantees its theoretical inadequacy.

Illusory solutions: the QALY

The same can be said of the second solution I want to consider. The quality-adjusted life year (QALY) is proposed as an ethical solution to the problems of rationing. One of its most prominent defenders, Alan Williams, explains the idea as follows.

> *'Commonsense tells us that in the face of scarcity we should use our limited resources in such a way that they do as much good as possible. In healthcare, "doing good" means improving people's life expectancy and the quality of their lives . . . The essence of the QALY concept is that effects on life expectancy and effects on quality of life are brought together in a single measure. . .' (Williams 1995, p. 222)*

Unlike Wall, Williams eschews neither rationality nor objectivity. The claim that 'we should . . . do as much good as possible' sounds like one of Wall's principles, but Williams attempts to provide a more precise definition of what 'doing good' in this context means. The idea of a 'QALY' is initially exciting because it offers the possibility of an objective measurement to determine what counts as 'the best thing' one could do in any given set of circumstances. In rationing, there will always be consequences which are 'unfortunate for someone or other' (op cit) but at least it becomes possible to make the best of a bad lot, once we know what this means: the 'best' outcome being the outcome that brings about the most QALYs.

The problems arise when we attempt to give some content to the concept of the QALY. Williams assumes that this can be done 'empirically':

> *'the empirical work involved in making the concept operational is concerned with eliciting the values that people attach to different health states . . .'*

In other words, to find out what is really most valuable, we ask people to tell us what, as a matter of fact, they value. This simply assumes a subjectivist theory of value: it takes it as read that people cannot be wrong about the values they attach to things. Williams may not be troubled by the fact that this is a huge assumption, totally without support in his work. He should perhaps be more troubled by the fact that, understood properly, it would render the whole project in which he is engaged meaningless. Firstly, if all value judgements are subjective, then there is no sense to asking what anyone 'ought' to do about anything, since we can have no basis for a rational debate about any practical question. If people share our subjective reactions then there is no need for a debate and if they don't then we can only hope to sway them, by non-rational persuasion, round to our way of thinking. So the attempt to discuss how the health service ought to be organised using rational, academic arguments is misguided, unless subjectivism about values is a false theory.

Secondly, it makes no sense to ask what 'we' value most, when 'we' refers to a group whose members disagree about values, both with one another and each member with herself, over time (since people change their minds about what they value). Each person can say 'what is valuable for me, now' (the fact that they might not be sure, and might have to give it a great deal of thought, should suggest that there is something wrong with the subjectivist assumption) but there is no intellectually defensible way to move from the activity of soliciting and recording such judgements to a view about what is 'really' valuable or 'most' valuable.

The similarities between the QALY approach and the easy solution start to emerge when we consider Williams' response to such problems (or rather, his dismissal of them, since he does not think that they are really problems for the QALY at all). He is fully aware that any policy maker using the QALY device to make rationing decisions would have to make decisions about whose values to count (since obviously it would not be possible to question every person affected by a policy) and how to move 'from individual values to group values'. He also acknowledges that there are distinct questions which the QALY cannot answer about how benefits are distributed, once we have discovered the 'amount' of benefits which accrue from specific health service activities (Williams 1995, p. 224).

Williams seems quite content to accept that there can be no determinate answer to such questions. As a health economist, it is 'not for him to say' how the device is employed in practice and he treats the flexibility of the QALY when it comes to answering such questions (meaning, its ability to leave any answer open when it comes to such questions) as one of its virtues:

> 'The QALY concept is extremely accommodating in this respect. In principle it can accept anybody's views about what is important in health-related quality of life, and anybody's views about the trade-off between length and quality of life.'

On the move 'from individual to group values' he says: 'there is nothing in the QALY approach which requires aggregation to be accomplished in any particular way.' He then describes distinct ways of arriving at the 'collective' view, following the soliciting of individual views, making it clear that a variety of different and incompatible 'collective' views could purport to be 'based on' the individual views expressed. Similarly, on the issue of the distribution of benefits: 'there is nothing in the QALY approach which requires QALYs to be used only in a maximizing context'. One might determine the 'collective' view in a way that did not involve 'QALY maximisation' as the 'collective prioritising rule'.

The theoretical adequacy of the QALY in determining the 'best' allocation of resources must surely be questioned, once we realise that it is compatible with many distinct, and mutually incompatible, methods for arriving at practical decisions. The objectivity of this approach is illusory, since there is no determinate answer to the question of how we organise the information acquired empirically; nor can there be any answer to the question of whether the views solicited in any empirical survey represent the 'right' answers, for the whole approach implicitly accepts that there are no right answers.

This same flexibility makes it useful to policy makers since, given the right method of aggregation, a wide variety of policies could be given 'justification' with reference to the QALY. The device is also very 'accommodating' to those who want to make 'priority setting' seem more rational since, in addition to its bogus 'objectivity' it successfully disguises the incommensurability of many of the values involved in decisions about the allocation of health resources. By insisting that people rank options, we assume that a ranking is intelligible: effectively, we make it a matter of necessity that all values must be commensurable. Thus, the problem of incommensurability is systematically ignored and it is assumed that it must always be in principle possible to make a rational choice between two options (a point which Wall rightly treated as obviously false). Williams' 'empirical' methods make decisions which can only be arbitrary appear non-arbitrary, by disguising the arbitrary origins of the so-called 'judgements' on which they are based.

These points aside, the QALY device assumes implicitly the legitimacy of the economic structure which determines scarcity, by taking as read every feature of social reality other than the health service. There are many determinants of the length and quality of life, but Williams only considers the effects of medical interventions. He states that 'in a resource-constrained system "cost" means "sacrifice"' (Williams 1995, p. 223), arguing that benefits given to one patient necessarily lead to benefits being foregone by others. As I have pointed out, something is only necessary given certain conditions and Williams chooses to examine no other features of the social world than medical services. This effectively assumes that every other feature of the economy is 'beyond question' or that it is not 'our' business to question it, because 'we' are concerned with healthcare policy. But there is no reason for human beings to bind themselves to thinking in categories arbitrarily dictated by the political structure as it is, as if thinking about healthcare means imagining oneself to be the 'minister responsible for healthcare' and imagining what one should do with one's limited budget (assuming that the possibility of persuading the Chancellor to give health a bit more is out of the question).

It is not clear that having an intelligent view about health means thinking of the health service in isolation from the rest of social reality, imagining 'other things are equal'. The ascription of causal efficacy to one feature of social reality is neither a naive nor a value-neutral activity. To say that spending in one area of the health service leads necessarily to shortages in another area is not to make a purely 'empirical' observation. Rather, Williams performs a thought-experiment in which he assumes that every other feature of the world is the same, except that the benefits which in fact went to one group of patients might instead have been allocated to a different group. Noting that in that case things would have been better for the second group and worse for the first, he concludes that the benefits enjoyed by the first group necessitated the sacrifices made by the second. But one might equally argue that increased salaries for the leaders of industry 'necessitated' the sacrifices made by the second group. For one can imagine a situation in which the first group enjoyed the same benefits and in which no sacrifices were made by the second group either, since the salaries of the rich were cut dramatically and the money saved was spent on the second group. It all depends on which counter-factual one chooses to think about and that in turn depends on one's political position. Williams' position, like that of any naive participant in the 'rationing' debate, is inherently reactionary.

Williams might perhaps respond to this by claiming that he is only being realistic, since the health service *is* a 'resource-constrained system'. This would be to miss the point. Which counter-factual one chooses to think about does not depend on how 'realistic' one is: as a matter of logic, to think about a counter-factual situation is to think about a situation which is not real. Unwillingness to think about radical changes in the organisation of social reality when trying to determine what is right or best reflects not realism but the unwillingness to admit any major differences between the way the world is and how it ought to be. It suggests the disposition to believe that the world is just about right as it is, that the social background to health service policy is morally uncontroversial.

Thus I am not complaining that the world is not 'perfect', in which case Williams would answer that we just have to make the best of it. My claim is that, when it comes to the type of decisions that Williams is most concerned to address, we have no way of determining what 'making the best of it' means. The assumption that there must be a defensible, determinate answer to questions about who should be allowed to suffer and die is false. To take a typical sort of discussion from the rationing debate, not only is it not obvious that we can find an acceptable rational answer to the question 'Should the elderly (who have worked all their lives, contributed to the system, etc.) be sacrificed for the sake of the very young (who have all their lives ahead of them, who are innocent, etc.)?' The very idea that we can do so is offensive nonsense and the attempt to construct devices or principles which enable people to make such decisions 'ethically' is an attempt to make nonsense of ethics. Why should the categories mentioned be capable of being fed into any calculation or decision making procedure, however sophisticated, which weighs their relative moral merit? Should society ever evolve beyond its present state of semi-barbarism, such questions will not be answered but rather abolished. Theory may be able to help this process, but only by addressing a general audience in the hope of encouraging critical thinking within the populace at large. Theorists who purport to be able to 'solve' our very specific and present problems only add to the moral and intellectual chaos of the modern world, by reassuring us that if we think about it in the right way, the unacceptable becomes acceptable. Viewed under the right light, phrased in the right language, the brutality and injustice inherent in any rationing procedure can, it seems, become rational and just.

The true function of 'ethical committees'

This brings us back to the question of the purpose of the activity of theorising and the assumptions theorists make about their role and audience. In the final chapter of *Life and Death: philosophical essays in biomedical ethics*, the influential American bioethicist Dan Brock comments on his experiences as 'staff philosopher' on a presidential commission whose remit was to study 'Ethical Problems in Medicine' and on various other committees, 'at both state and national level' (Brock 1993, p. 408). While Brock thinks that in philosophy generally 'what is important is that other scholars are persuaded by their own assessment of one's arguments and evidence' (ibid, p. 413), he sees the ultimate target audience of applied philosophy as 'policy makers'. Thus philosophers who are not 'fortunate enough to have the opportunity to use their analytical and critical skills at influential points in the policy process' (ibid, p. 415) are described as 'academics just hoping that an occasional policy-maker might read their scholarly journal articles' (p. 409).

This view about the target audience certainly should, in Brock's view, influence how one approaches the work in hand.

Philosophers should write with 'a more realistic understanding of the constraints of political reality', avoiding the natural temptation to 'set agendas that are unrealistically wide' (pp. 414–15). The British philosopher Michael Lockwood writes on 'the prospect of a philosopher chairing a government inquiry' that:

> 'It is gratifying to think that the powers that be recognise and value the philosopher's peculiar kind of expertise; it is gratifying also that, for once, philosophy might impinge on the real world.' (Lockwood 1985, p. 55)

Lockwood immediately clarifies what it means for philosophy to 'impinge on the real world'. It means 'that Parliamentary legislation might be guided by philosophical considerations' (op cit). His only reservations about this idea concern the fact that 'philosophers disagree with one another'. This is an important point, but not quite (or at least not only) for the reasons Lockwood gives. He wonders:

> 'whether the philosophically trained chairman of a government committee is providing the right sort of philosophical guidance [since] . . . the philosopher chairing the committee is likely to be the only philosophically trained person there; things he or she might say, the contentiousness of which would be immediately apparent to a fellow member of the profession, are thus likely to go unchallenged.' (op cit)

We might feel that when it comes to the formation of government policy 'better no philosophy at all . . . than wrong-headed philosophy'. He adds two statements which, when taken together, are very revealing. He says that in his view 'almost every philosopher' would relish the chance to advise a government inquiry and he concludes from this that 'the Platonic conception of the philosopher king dies hard'. What all these points take for granted is the idea that the presence of a philosopher on a government committee means that *philosophy* is influencing policy. (The 'philosopher king' analogy suggests that the influence is direct and significant.) Lockwood's reservation states the concern that the philosophy should be good philosophy (and the difficulty in determining what this is, given the controversial nature of the subject). But this assumption is, to say the least, questionable. It is reminiscent of the idea that by making a poor person Prime Minister, we ensure that the interests of the poor are represented at the highest level (rather than, instead, making one poor person no longer poor): it completely disregards the influence of context on human thought and behaviour. Not only this, it assumes an extremely dubious model of policy determination.

To take the second point first, it might make sense to speak of philosophy influencing policy if a Platonic philosopher king made every policy decision. I think it would still be false to speak of philosophy totally determining policy, since while the king might do his best to form every policy on the basis of moral reasoning, he would inevitably be influenced by other factors and his reasoning might often be flawed. Nonetheless, philosophy would in this case be a strong influence. The correct model of policy formation, however, in no way resembles the idea of an individual following certain reasoning processes which directly determine a decision. A two-level model is still far too simplistic, but it will serve to convey my point.

Imagine an overall process whose results are determined at one level by a governing process G, which selects between an indeterminate number of other, secondary processes, A, B, C . . . to bring about the final results (the results being certain decisions or policies). The methods of the secondary processes are different and often opposed to one another. The governing process has its own methods for selecting which of the secondary processes to use, to bring about its desired results. Its methods are also often in conflict with those of many of the secondary processes: were process C, for instance, the governing process, it would never select process B for any purposes whatsoever, but process G sometimes will. It would be misleading to claim that, on the occasion when process C is selected, the methods of that process determine, or even in any real sense influence, the overall process. For process C was only selected because in this instance the results it promised to deliver were judged, by the standards of process G, to be desirable.

Now suppose that process C is philosophy. Does philosophy really, in any meaningful sense, influence policy if some other process determines when the views of philosophers will be called on and which philosopher will be called? When philosophers advise those whom Lockwood calls 'the powers that be' they are not chosen in accordance with philosophical criteria, nor do such criteria influence the choice of issue on which they are requested to speak: the philosophers' remit is determined by political, not philosophical considerations. To speak, in such circumstances, of philosophy 'influencing' the political process, without giving any consideration to why certain philosophers are asked to speak on only certain specific issues, is to promote a wilfully naive picture of the nature of government. Can anyone seriously claim to wonder why the US government called on Dan Brock (whose political position is strongly influenced by the liberal contractualist thinking of John Rawls) to comment on specific questions in medical ethics before making certain policy decisions, but then failed to procure advice on the ethics of war from anarchist professor Robert Paul Wolff (whose academic philosophical credentials are at least as impressive as those of Brock) before coming to a decision about whether to invade Iraq?

Even ignoring the significance of the process of selection, those philosophers who are selected take on a political role when they find themselves in the 'real world of politics'. Brock himself freely admits this. Indeed, the whole point of his chapter is to discuss the dilemmas this creates. Brock states that 'the different goals of academic scholarship and public policy call in turn for different virtues and behaviour in their practitioners' (Brock 1993, p. 409). In philosophy 'nothing is to be immune from question and criticism . . . Whether the results are unpopular or in conflict with conventional or authoritative views, determining the truth to the best of one's abilities is the goal' (op cit).

This commitment to the truth comes under 'a variety of related pressures' when philosophers 'enter the policy domain' (pp. 409–10). To voice 'extreme, unconventional, or radical views', simply because one believes, on the basis of reasoned arguments, they are true, is to 'risk using up one's credibility and to risk not being heard, or even losing the opportunity to speak, on other occasions when one might have a significant impact' (p. 413). In the new context, philosophers 'must shift their primary commitment from knowledge and truth to the policy consequences of what they do' (p. 410). Brock gives an example from his own experience which supposedly illustrates why it is their moral responsibility to do so. As staff philosopher to a presidential commission, Brock's 'bosses' (his word) were commissioners 'who were political appointees out of the office of the president' (not philosophers):

> 'The Commissioners had the final word on what our reports would say. Thus . . . my own views . . . would only have any effect if I was able to persuade other staff members . . . and in turn the Commissioners, of them.' (ibid, p. 410)

As a result:

> 'The goal often became to persuade or even to manipulate others in order to reach a desired outcome instead of a common search for the truth.' (p. 411)

The one example Brock gives to justify this concerns euthanasia. He believes there is no morally important distinction between killing and letting die and that stopping life-sustaining treatment is killing – though often justified killing. He defends this view with admirable clarity in other chapters of the same text. However, he did not press this line to the commissioners because, it seems, he knew that they would disagree. Apart from 'using up' his 'credibility', Brock feared that by pressing his position he might have convinced his political bosses that stopping life-sustaining treatment is morally wrong. This would entail their only partially following his reasoning, but rather than risk this, Brock decided to let them go on in their 'confusions', letting them believe what they believed already: that there is a morally important distinction between killing and letting die and that stopping life-sustaining treatment is a form of 'letting die', not of killing. By 'playing a little fast and loose with the truth' (p. 412) Brock aimed to bring about consequences which, according to his own moral views, were the best ones for patients.

Brock states that if philosophers sit on such committees, this is how they should behave. It is astonishing that he does not give more serious consideration to the claim that they *should not* sit on such committees. For, on his own account of the proceedings, he was participating in fraud. Unlike Brock, my father (a former dock worker) has never been asked to sit on a government committee to discuss bioethics, the reason being that he lacks Brock's academic status. Brock brings to the process a certain academic credibility: he bears the title of 'philosopher' and a (well-deserved) reputation for being a 'good' philosopher with 'relevant' expertise. What, however, do these words signify? What message does their association with policy process convey?

Brock admits that philosophers are not 'moral authorities': being a philosopher does not mean you are thereby more likely to know the right answers on moral questions. Lockwood's point is important here. Since philosophers disagree with each other, often radically, it would be a mistake to think that by asking a philosopher for his or her views on any particular moral question, you are more likely to receive the correct answer than if you asked a dock worker. (Recall my earlier point about the difference between a 'pharmacist' and an 'ethicist'.) Philosophers are valued not for their conclusions, but for the methods by which they reach their conclusions. It is how one approaches a problem that distinguishes one as a philosopher. Yet Brock admits that the philosophical method (what he describes (p. 409) as philosophers' 'academic ways') must be the first thing to go when one enters the 'policy-making process'. One attempts to manipulate others to agree with one's own conclusions, whatever they are, by whatever means one can, even when this means 'playing a little fast and loose with the truth'. So Brock brings the *name* of philosophy into the political process, but not its *methods*.

How would he react to this analogy? A civil engineer of excellent reputation is employed by a large corporation to act as 'resident civil engineer', advising on a variety of building projects, and is listed as such in all the documentation associated with the projects. Should it be discovered that this person only ever gave advice on aesthetic aspects of the projects in question and so did not make use of his relevant skills as part of the work he did for the corporation, would Brock feel he made an 'ethical' use of his title and reputation? Brock's claim, then, that philosophers use their 'analytical and critical skills' to 'improve' the policy process, producing 'real and significant benefits' (p. 415), seems somewhat lacking in support from his own account. He says that philosophers might help to 'widen the agenda' (p. 414) but he gives no example to illustrate what he might mean: would the ultra-conservative philosopher Roger Scruton help to widen the agenda in the same way that the left-of-centre Bernard Williams would? We all, I think, have a good idea as to what philosophers (and other academics) really contribute to such proceedings. They serve to foster the illusion that decisions of state are the result of impartial, objective reasoning 'informed' by 'experts'. They bestow academic credibility on policies and (most importantly) on the whole policy-forming procedure, making it subsequently harder for others – particularly those lacking academic standing – to criticise the policies. They convey a bogus sense of authority, 'the work of the favoured theorists thus functioning as another stick in the already impressive armoury of the powerful' (Loughlin 1994a, p. 47).

The mythology of liberalism

The idea that the proper role of applied philosophy is to 'influence politicians and the powerful' can therefore be questioned. Even those few philosophers who get the chance to make recommendations to the state find that the key philosophical virtues of intellectual honesty and logical consistency are the first things that have to be abandoned if they are to retain their 'credibility' as political advisors. How much less sense, then, does it make for the majority of theorists to go on 'hoping that the occasional policy maker will read their scholarly journal articles' (assuming Brock is right and that is indeed what they are doing)? Governments make decisions in terms of many factors, few of which have anything to do with a concern to do the 'right' thing. If they did want to know what was the right thing, it is surely overwhelmingly unlikely they would base their views on the contents of academic journals.[24] If philosophical debate has any practical purpose then it is not to make direct recommendations to the powers that be about which policies to adopt.

This raises serious questions about the presuppositions of applied philosophy, particularly for the work of bioethicists. Discussing how 'we' could make healthcare policy – and indeed society generally – more 'rational' and/or 'ethical' (suggesting that 'we' could 'realistically' make this or that change and that 'we should' do so) presupposes that the relevant social and political forces are under 'our' control. However, the collective 'we' assumed here is fictional: those who in fact influence policy are not party to the debate and will not be influenced by the sort of thinking that constitutes its essential character. The very idea that they might be derives from an ideological assumption: indeed, it is rooted in a way of conceiving of the social world that is so deep-seated and seems so natural to our pre-reflective consciousness that it deserves to be viewed as part of the *mythology* of contemporary political culture.

Many of the classical texts in liberal political philosophy describe a situation in which rational human beings, in a presocial state ('state of nature'), come together to create the conditions of social life. (Hobbes 1968, Locke 1967, Rousseau 1947). On the basis of rational deliberations to determine what is to their mutual advantage, they agree on rules by which each person should be governed and they construct a state to enforce those rules. From that point onwards they no longer live in a state of nature: they are now part of 'civil society' and bound by its laws and norms. Philosophers have held a variety of views concerning the precise role descriptions of such scenarios have in political thinking. Clearly they do not describe the true historical origins of human society, so it is instead often claimed that they bring out certain key logical points about our social and political obligations. It strikes me that they are more fundamental to our thinking, even, than that. The scenario sketched is more like what historian Roger Griffin (1993) would call a 'myth'. A myth in this sense is an idea or image that motivates behaviour and determines how we think of ourselves and our relationship with the world (ibid, p. 27). It is an ideal which inspires emotional commitment, for which some of its adherents might even be prepared to die. For instance, the 'mythic core' of fascist ideology concerns the idea of rebirth: persons who adopt this ideology see themselves as part of a community that has been crushed by hostile forces but is on the point of rising like the phoenix to meet its destiny (ibid, p. 26). We are more comfortable thinking about the myths of alien philosophies, such as fascism, than we are thinking about the myths which underlie the dominant ideology in our own culture. (Especially since that ideology tends to frown on the mythological.)

The image of a society created by free rational agents, whose rules and structure are determined by the consent of all its members for their mutual advantage, may be seen to form the 'mythic core' of liberal democratic ideology. It is certainly an idea that many find inspiring. The state, on this view, exists to represent the collective will of those agents. Thus it makes perfect sense to engage the state in rational debate and to assume that by doing so one is helping to determine policy: any rational agent could propose a policy and if it can be demonstrated really to be advantageous then it surely will be adopted.

Griffin thinks of myths as 'non-rational' and therefore not susceptible to rational criticism. They are not supposed to be true: they are simply ideas to inspire us. This may be so, but we surely can assess rationally the decision to construe one's relationship with one's own society in terms of a particular myth. If doing so causes us to distort the nature of social reality, then doing so is irrational. Unless we construe contemporary democracies in terms of the liberal myth, much of the debate in bioethics makes no sense. Suppose we think of the state not as the expression of rational collective choice but, as William Godwin put it, as a 'brute engine' (Godwin 1985). By this Godwin meant a social mechanism whose behaviour is suscep-tible to analysis (like any mechanism) and is sometimes, there-fore, predictable, but which does not display features of rational agency. In that case, attempting to influence its behaviour by constructing moral arguments makes about as much sense as King Canute's tide control strategy. Surely we can ask whether or not Godwin's image comes closer to representing the truth about our present situation than the central myth of liberalism – and, indeed, conclude that it does? But in that case the very activity of discussing bioethics (at least as these discussions are most commonly conducted) is irrational.

The problems this creates, however, are not restricted to bioethics: they affect the whole character of political conversation in today's liberal democracies. When thinking about political issues, we tend to imagine ourselves in the position of a policy maker; we think about what it would be best to do in that position and conclude that this is what should be done. Unlike other types of evaluative discourse (for instance, a conversation between a husband and wife about which school it would be best for them to send their children to), the conclusion that 'we should' do X has no direct practical significance, since it does not determine the behaviour of those who are in fact making the decision under discussion. We talk in this way because the mythology of liberal democratic society suggests that the decisions of the democratic state are really 'our' decisions, that we 'the public' (a collection of free, rational agents) determine policy via such a process of deliberation. But as we have seen, these ideas have no bearing whatsoever on reality. Does any serious analysis of the decisions of those in power make reference to such ideas? Of course, public opinion is a factor they consider but it is for the most part not formed by rational processes, it is easily manipulated and it is only one factor in any case.

We can of course talk about what specific persons, including leaders, 'should do', morally criticising them if they fail to act as we judge that they should. If this were all that political thinking involved then we would be logically obliged to limit our critical faculties to choosing between the options presented to us by the political parties: we could not criticise the system itself, nor could we attack features of the social structure that form the background to particular decisions; the context of the decisions would have to be simply taken as read. Some philosophical conservatives might accept this, dismissing not only bioethics but all attempts to criticise the prevailing social order as self-deluded 'rationalism' (Oakeshott 1962).

If rationality is to have any role in political debate (if we are to avoid the irrationalism criticised above) then we have to be clear about the limits and presuppositions of our discussion.

Otherwise our words will implicitly deny that those limits exist and will form part of the pretence that we live in an idealised democracy. This pretence may legitimately be described as a 'false consciousness': we are operating with a false picture of our relationship to the world which determines the nature of our language and neutralises its ability to solve real problems. It is at this level that philosophy can make a contribution.

Philosophers should realise that their work will have little or no impact on how the powerful make their decisions. There is no point trying to be a philosopher king. If they want to make an impact on the 'real world' they should attempt to address a general audience with the aim of enabling people to question common assumptions and traditional ways of conceptualising problems. Instead of constructing moral codes which over-simplify social life, they should try to pass on what skills they have to individuals struggling to make sense of a complex and brutish world. *We do not need sets of principles for doctors, nurses and managers: we need reflective people able to analyse problems, aware of their limitations and able to distinguish sense from nonsense.* While this may seem a less glamorous role for the philosopher than that envisaged by many of the ethicists whose arguments I have considered in this section, it is at once a more realistic and a more challenging and ambitious one.

As noted in the opening comments of this book, philosophy is for anyone sane enough to feel the need for it. In Part Four, I will attempt to spell out the ways in which philosophy, as so construed, can make a real impact upon the lives of people working in the health service and elsewhere. We will see that philosophy is not sufficient to solve the broader social problems that have been considered here, but that its absence ensures that these problems cannot be adequately addressed, nor even identified and adequately characterised. Thus the promotion of philosophy is a necessary step on the road to moral progress. If philosophy is to make a difference to people's lives its role must be to arm them against those who would lead them where they should not go, who would bury their ability to reason beneath layers of stifling rhetoric. Good applied philosophy will always be primarily reactive and critical, attacking ideologies that peddle false pictures of the world and bringing out the ideological commitments in common ways of discussing problems. Significant social change can only come from changes in social consciousness. As Godwin observed, a reflective, critical populace is a prerequisite for meaningful social change. Anything philosophers can do to encourage critical thought is therefore a worthwhile contribution to the struggle.

Part Four

Moral education in an irrational world

Chapter 7

Agent-centred ethics and the nature of value

So where have we come to – and how did we get here? If the reader is new to philosophy, and if she has approached the arguments of the preceding pages with openness, attentiveness and clarity of mind, then she may by this stage be feeling somewhat disconcerted. Instead of finding solutions to the problems of the organisation of health services we have, so far, discovered instead a whole series of problems for the very project of finding solutions to those problems. If my account of the context of the problems under discussion has been sufficiently clear and vivid, and if my criticisms of the various solutions on offer have been appropriately detailed and penetrating, then the reader should by now have a strong sense of just how difficult it is to say anything about these problems that is at once true and worth saying. The approaches of management theory and bioethics do not work and cannot work. Indeed, we can only begin to think seriously and effectively about the issues at stake when we free ourselves of the assumptions behind these approaches – assumptions which seem only too natural to us and whose rejection has implications which potentially extend far beyond the issues surrounding the management and delivery of health services. We need to think carefully about the way we approach practical problems, if we are not to commit ourselves to pictures of our lives and practices which effectively undermine our best efforts to make progress. If by now the reader feels the need for a different approach then something has been achieved and the pages filled so far have not been wasted paper.

That is not to say that the reader will by now be feeling 'satisfied'. Too many academic books today evaluate arguments and conclusions in terms of how 'satisfying' they are. Like the use of the word 'positive', this smacks of thoughtless consumerism: the reader is a 'customer' who wants to be 'satisfied' by a 'positive' outcome. If the reader craves satisfaction she can seek out a romantic novel with a guaranteed happy ending. If she is seeking a truly educational experience then she must be prepared to be challenged, frustrated, upset, even deeply disturbed by what she finds. Given the state of the world, a book about 'ethics' which is at all realistic should leave the reader feeling deeply dissatisfied. A sense of dissatisfaction necessarily attends the development of a critical awareness of one's environment. It may even lead to a slightly uncomfortable sense of isolation as one realises oneself to be engaged in a process of reasoning about a world whose nature is determined largely by forces that are neither rational nor morally conscionable.

At least she cannot say she has been misled. I began by offering not a 'solution' in the conventional sense but a vantage point, a place to start thinking in a clear and honest way about the reality that one hopes to affect, and a method of reasoning in terms of which to approach problems with rigour and intellectual honesty. The practice of questioning fundamental assumptions can be profoundly disorientating – like the feeling of looking down and discovering that, where before you had believed yourself to be on solid ground, you are in fact on a narrow beam and the ground is somewhere out of sight, far below.[1] This sense of disorientation is only exacerbated if one has worked most of one's life in the sort of context where the questioning of fundamental assumptions is discouraged (either explicitly or by the sheer pressure the demands of the job exert upon one's intellectual energy). Yet the alternative is much worse: to refuse to examine the conditions of one's life for fear that one may not like what one finds. Only once we have gone through the process of thinking our way out from our immediate situation, to develop an overview of that situation and all the factors which affect it, and only once we have overcome the sense of intellectual vertigo that this can create, can we focus back on the immediate and claim to see it for what it is. And only then can we begin to develop adequate responses to the problems which confront us, since we cannot hope to solve problems whose true nature we do not understand.

So far, then, we have reached a vantage point. We have some idea of the true nature and causes of the problems under discussion: we can locate them in relation to other questions about the structure of the society in which the health service must function and the ideological shifts which are reshaping that society, transforming in the process the thinking and practices of all its public services. We know something of the conceptual lie of the land and, armed with this knowledge, we can start to think seriously about what it might mean to attempt to manage 'ethically' in the context of such a service. What, if anything, can a work of theory say that will actually be helpful to the decent and intelligent reader attempting to practise in as civilised and rational a manner as possible within a social world infected with irrationality and arbitrary brutality? To return to the 'murder novel' analogy of Chapter 1, the attentive reader will not be mystified by this question since many of the components of the answer are there already, either explicitly, in what has actually been stated, or implicitly, in what can be deduced from what has been stated. To move forward it is necessary to take cognisance of what has gone before, to note what it rules out and to identify whatever remains as that which it is possible to assert.

The story so far

I began by identifying the approach of the book in terms of a particular style of thinking: philosophy is the practice of conceptual analysis; it is a method of thinking which exposes fundamental assumptions and hidden commitments in the inferences we make and even in the questions we think it pertinent to ask. Only by use of this method of analysis can we begin to understand, and so hope to shape, the forces which determine how we live our lives and so it is an essential component of the practical thinking of any free person. I then considered the various philosophical theories concerning the nature of moral thinking. Theories like deontology and consequentialism are the staple of applied moral philosophy and they do help us to identify the different types of moral consideration which any situation may present. However, our intuitions about what we should do in any specific case may be in part determined by features of the context which are unique. Furthermore, we can only assess the relative merits of the various moral theories by developing sound moral intuitions, so the debate in moral philosophy, if it is to have any sensible resolution, must turn its attention to the question of what it means to develop good intuitions and how in practice we are to acquire them. Unfortunately, the most well-known form of the doctrine known as 'intuitionism' was found to be unsound. The claim to know 'by intuition' that certain basic moral propositions are true was seen to embody claims that are questionable on both logical and epistemological grounds and the doctrine was therefore unhelpful in determining the proper conduct of a human life in any practical context.

At this point the search for a philosophically adequate account of moral reasoning was put on hold, in order to consider an approach to evaluation in health services management that eschews philosophical methods. The attempt to develop a so-called 'science' of management was seen to embody a basic logical confusion concerning the meaning of evaluative terms and its popularity was accounted for in terms of its compatibility with consumerist ideology. The new 'management theory' was found guilty of the dual sins of formalism and dogmatism. Its exponents attempt to reduce human practices to sets of principles which, when followed, will automatically lead to a 'quality' outcome in any complex area of practice and they refuse to consider the possibility that their basic assumptions are incorrect – indeed, they refuse even to give an honest account of these assumptions. This 'management theory' turns out to be not only nonsense but dangerous, ideologically inspired nonsense which threatens to destroy values that are essential to anything that can qualify as a morally acceptable health service. The ideologues of this approach to management are part of a broader movement that bids us to think about every feature of social life in terms of the language and concepts of market economics and the effects of this conceptual shift are rarely explained, let alone debated within the culture it proposes to 'transform'.

To resist or even to question this movement, we need to do philosophy. We need the intellectual skill to expose and criticise conceptualisations of our lives and practices implicit within the messages we receive and to reject those which we have been given no good reasons to accept. To explain and defend the role of philosophy in practical thinking, it was necessary to break down certain common dichotomies: between the practical and the theoretical, between reason and feelings and between intuition and rationality. Theories represent the ways in which we organise experiences, the conceptual maps in terms of which we negotiate our world: so the person who says 'I am not interested in theory' is someone whose thinking is conditioned by theories whose influence he fails to understand or even to recognise. Similarly 'feelings' and 'reason' cannot be understood in isolation from each other. Feelings are attitudes which presuppose certain beliefs and entail dispositions to behave in certain ways. Thus we can explain people's behaviour in terms of the way they feel and we can have good reasons for the way we feel. Reasoning is an activity which characterises a rational agent and to possess rationality is to be disposed to organise one's experiences in certain ways. The implications of this for the relationship between 'intuitions' and 'rationality' were hinted at and will be developed in more detail shortly.

Unfortunately, much of the current debate in 'bioethics' was found to embody the very assumptions about theory and practice which must be abandoned. It is the 'repair manual' school of applied philosophy, since it presupposes a characterisation of the context of the problems it discusses which it fails to defend, or even to subject to serious philosophical scrutiny, and then sets about 'solving' those problems via the direct application of ideas or principles derived from moral philosophy.

As a result much of the work in this area is, like that of the management theorists, characterised by dogmatism and formalism. Even if it were possible to devise a set of values, goals or principles that were somehow definitive of 'ethical practice', the gap between these ideas (be they devised by 'management scientists' or philosophers) and behaviour in the unique and complex situations moral agents face could only ever be bridged by the intuitive reactions of the agent, so the claim that we can 'apply' such ideas to help secure an 'ethical' outcome is misleading. In any case, when the nature of a social context is determined largely by irrational or non-rational factors, it makes no sense to attempt to affect it via the direct application of rational principles. So for the bioethical enterprise to be possible, society must be construed as essentially rational in nature. The influence of this idea was traced to a picture of the social world embedded so deeply in the thinking of a liberal political culture that it must be treated as part of that culture's mythology. It is because of the idea's mythological status that its influence (and evident falsity) remains largely unrecognised. Far from encouraging critical thinking, by its very existence bioethics encourages unthinking acceptance of the dominant myths in our own society.

This may appear to lead us to an impasse but, as noted above, the way forward is implied by what has gone before. The discussions of moral theory (Chapter 2) and the role of feelings in moral reasoning (Chapter 5) brought out the need for a defensible conception of moral intuition, but also the inadequacy of any form of intuitionism which claims we can base our moral thinking upon intuitive knowledge of certain propositions (or of the 'non-natural properties' to which these propositions supposedly make reference). But this is not what most of us mean by the word 'intuition' anyway. We mean something more like an inclination, a sense of something: to have an intuition is to be instinctively disposed to do certain things and not others or to believe certain things and not others. To say that something is 'intuitively wrong' is to say it just feels wrong: we are instinctively disposed to reject it. Thus a more defensible form of intuitionism is possible if intuition is construed not as knowledge of basic moral propositions but the possession of fundamental *rational dispositions*. Our concept of rationality is a practical concept: to be a rational agent is to be disposed to react in certain ways, to treat certain types of experience as reasons to form certain conclusions. Even the tendency to construe one's experiences as experiences of an independent world was seen to be a disposition in this sense and, what is more, it is a disposition that is definitive of one's status as rational. This suggests the direction we must take in pursuit of an adequate theory of moral thinking, one which avoids the pitfalls of irrationalism but also takes full note of the role of feelings in the formation of moral judgements.

It is necessary to make the concept of rational agency the primary object of philosophical inquiry, to ask not 'what principles or rules should we live by?' or 'what outcomes should we aim to bring about?' but rather 'what sort of dispositions should we develop?' and 'how do we go about developing them?' The failings of management theory (Part Two) and bioethics (Chapter 6) also usher us along this avenue of inquiry. The formalism and the dogmatism of these approaches are closely related: because these theorists attempt to answer questions of the former sort (about the principles or rules of good conduct or about the sort of outcome it is rational to aim for) they are forced to ignore or deny those features of the world which make a clear and informative answer to these questions impossible.

The contexts in which people must make decisions are too diverse, too unpredictable and frequently too ambiguous to allow for the meaningful application of any set of principles or rules of conduct in the resolution of real problems. There will always be a 'gap' between this sort of theory and practice, which it will be necessary for practitioners to bridge by supplying their own intuitive responses: so it is these responses (not the theoretical devices employed) which in fact determine decisions. Unless theory can affect the intuitions of moral agents, it can have no meaningful influence on practice in any area. Real problems are not solved in books: they are solved by people in real situations. Words on a page have no causal efficacy unless they effect a change in those who read them, influencing their outlook on life, the way in which they are disposed to think about practical problems – their 'mentality' in the most general sense of this term. We must address ourselves to the nature of moral agency: the role of theory (if theorising is to be an activity we have any good reason to engage in) must be to produce the right people to face the world and this requires thinking carefully about the sort of people we want around and (perhaps more importantly) that we want to be.

Moral knowledge and human flourishing

To approach moral problems in this way is to adopt an agent-centred position in ethics. This approach is frequently associated with the work of Aristotle.[2] For Aristotle moral knowledge was practical in nature: it was concerned primarily with *knowing how* to live well, rather than with *knowing that* certain propositions were true, and moral life concerned the development of the virtues, meaning the right moral dispositions to enable human 'flourishing'. To 'flourish' is to become a good instance of one's kind, so the central question of moral philosophy becomes: how does one become a good person? How do we acquire the right sort of intuitive reactions to equip us to face the many and diverse situations that life may present?

In many situations, questions about what we should do are unclear and it is often the case that no formal characterisation of the situation suggests a determinate answer. It is unrealistic to hope that social contexts will become more straightforward, so it is unrealistic to hope for a theory that will directly determine good practice. People will always be in the predicament of 'plumping' for an answer and often the best we can hope for is that we will have the right sort of people doing the 'plumping'.[3] If we can have good people making decisions then the outcomes are more likely to be better. That is not to say that such people will be infallible: even when rational, sincere people make sound judgements, the outcome in an unpredictable and irrational context can be a poor one. Indeed, it may often be the case that there is no right decision, that the context leaves so little room for manoeuvre that any decision made is inadequate and arbitrary. Even in such cases, it is better to have intelligent people with moral integrity making decisions. One of the intellectual skills a good decision maker must possess is the ability to identify those situations where what should be done cannot be done because of certain features of the context in which he must practise. A professional population made up of thinkers such as this has within it the capacity to change the context of its practice for the better, while a population lacking such thinkers can only make things worse, ensuring that the context does not change and helping to perpetuate the dominant myths about it.

The desire for an infallible method is symptomatic of the formalistic attitudes which must be given up: if we cannot have a theory which gives us all 'the answers' we at least want a set of rules to learn which can automatically lead to the correct answers. This desire is so strong that some theorists are prepared to define the right answers as whatever answers one arrives at given that one follows the 'correct' procedures[4] (hence the fondness for 'ethical codes' in some areas of practice). Such attitudes betray intellectual immaturity. They represent the desire to avoid responsibility for one's own decisions by deferring to some 'impersonal' mechanism. (The fact that the mechanism has a human inventor is conveniently overlooked.)

As we saw in Chapter 2, the discovery that this is not possible can lead to the wholesale rejection of rationality on the part of some thinkers. The realisation that there are very few certainties in life, that the truth is often difficult to discover and that most serious questions are inherently controversial leads some theorists fairly directly to the conclusion that the truth is impossible to find and that rationality is therefore redundant. The move from the rejection of a simplistic form of rationalism (formalism) to some extreme form of anti-rationalism (such as postmodernism) reflects the implicit assumption that we should not have to think for ourselves. What both these extremes have in common is the failure to come to terms with one's own fallibility in the context of a complex, independent and often brutal world. The rejection of reason accomplishes the reintroduction of something akin to infallibility via the back door: if there is no sense in seeking the truth then we are each free to choose between the different versions of the truth on offer and no-one is in a position to tell us we are wrong.

The genuine sense of outrage that one detects in the writings of many contemporary anti-rationalists is reminiscent of a child who cannot forgive her parents for failing to be superhuman. We must experience a sense of horror at the stupidity and barbarity of the modern social world if we are not to live in a state of perpetual delusion, but we need to get over that shock – we need to grow up. The mature response is not to complain bitterly that one has been 'deceived' or 'betrayed' by the claims of 'reason'.

('Reason' never claimed to be sufficient to civilise humanity: certain *people* may have made such claims on behalf of 'reason' because their own reasoning was *flawed*. Specifically, they suffered from an insufficiently *realistic* view of the social world.) Rather, it is to learn how to live with the fact that there is no reliable map to direct us through life: we have to build up our own map as we go along and we must be prepared constantly to revise it. What we should be looking for in a work of theory is a demonstration of the skills necessary to help us in this task. We should be striving to become the sort of people who are up to the job. Intellectual life does not even begin until we recognise and accept the enormity of the challenge this presents.

It is sometimes claimed that the road to hell is paved with good intentions. I am not sure what we are supposed to conclude from this. Not, presumably, that the road to heaven is paved with bad intentions. We need to recognise the inherent imperfection (indeed, often the straightforward evil) of the modern social world, without giving way to absolute despair or descending into total irrationalism. The world is imperfect and our reasoning is imperfect, but that does not mean we can do without reasoning: we need it all the more. The alternative to thinking in a clear and disciplined way about how to live well is to have to face the same world without the benefit of such discipline, to allow one's thinking and one's reactions to be determined by factors one has waived the right to understand. The alternative to putting our trust in people with good motivations and trained in making sound judgements is to put our trust in people who lack such motivation and training. What is required, in health services management, in clinical practice, in education and in every area of professional and social life, is not more formalistic thinkers trained to memorise sets of rules and to parrot whatever is the currently fashionable jargon in their field. We have enough of those already. Instead we need a few more decent human beings, in possession of good intellectual instincts, able to analyse situations, to think honestly and critically, and with the courage and confidence to challenge nonsense and dogma. The key practical questions, and the key theoretical questions, are therefore the same: how do we get such people, how do we improve our own skills in these respects, and how do we ensure that more of these people are around? At least two of these are questions of moral education, so it is to that subject that I now want to turn.

Moral autonomy versus 'inculcatory' approaches

Much of the work in the field of moral education concerns the moral development of 'young people', although only the least astute contributors assume that 'education' means something that happens to us at the beginning of our lives and which we get over and done with by the time we have 'grown up'. While there are obvious practical reasons why many educators and theorists of education focus their efforts and attention on the young, fortunately for our present purposes this is by no means an essential feature of the debate about the underlying philosophical questions in the area. The day we decide we can stop learning, declaring that we know 'all that we need to know', is the day we stop growing as human beings. Far from suggesting intellectual maturity, this betrays stagnation: it is the decision to stop living a full human life, to switch on to automatic pilot and to allow the person one eventually becomes to be determined by a form of psychological inertia.

In ethics (and in life generally, since 'ethics' concerns the conduct of our lives in the broadest terms) the most important things we have to learn are not specific facts but general habits of thought and behaviour and it is just as important to maintain the right habits as it is to acquire them in the first place. As has been suggested (and will be expanded upon below), the most important habit we need to maintain as rational creatures is the habit of honest, critical thought: as fallible beings it is essential that we remain open to the possibility that what we have so far taken for granted is in some important respect misguided. If we lose this habit, if we cease to be open to new arguments concerning the validity of our own assumptions, then we have lost our critical capacities and with them the ability to learn – from experience, from the sincere and well-intentioned criticisms of others, indeed from anything at all. In that case we have become stupid dogmatists, intellectually and emotionally dead, like the 'grandes personnes' whose ranks Antoine de Saint-Exupéry (1981) was rightly determined never to join. Complacency is the enemy of intellectual life itself. Thinking, like breathing, is not a task one should ever hope to have completed.

In what follows I intend to present two of the key approaches to moral education. My characterisation of these approaches will be very brief, and tailored specifically to our present concerns. For a fuller introduction to these approaches I recommend the work of Wringe (1998a, b) with whom I am substantially in sympathy.[5] Wringe argues that there is something of the truth in each approach but that each is, in itself, inadequate. He argues further that an understanding of the Aristotelian concept of virtue provides the basis for an approach which incorporates what is worthwhile in each but avoids their respective pitfalls. At the heart of Wringe's criticisms is a conception of human reasoning which takes seriously the notion of realism with regard to value: we have the capacity to get it right or wrong when it comes to questions of how to live and practise and this is a capacity we possess as *human beings*, not merely as members of particular cultural or professional groups. The significance of these claims will hopefully become clearer in the light of the discussion of the alternatives.

The first of the two approaches treats the goal of moral education as:

> '*to promote moral reasoning leading, in successful cases, to that moral autonomy which would enable individuals to discover and, presumably, pursue their own considered version of the good life.*' (Wringe 1998b, p. 278)

To achieve this goal, discussions led by a 'neutral chairperson' (op cit) are advocated as a way of encouraging students to develop their reasoning skills. Wringe notes that there are serious 'practical and theoretical' problems for this approach. It is by no means clear why such discussions should lead to morally desirable conclusions or behaviour.

'The very discussion of moral issues may also suggest that well established and perfectly sound moral assumptions are, in fact, matters of doubt or even of taste and personal opinion, particularly if the discussion is inconclusive, confused or ineptly handled.' (Wringe 1998a, p. 226)

This outcome strikes me as built into the design of the whole approach. It is one thing for a group of people to engage in honest dialogue with the shared goal of discovering the truth about some important matter. It is quite a different thing to set up a tutor as a 'neutral chairperson' and to encourage a debate whose goal is to enable students to discover and defend their own 'version' of the truth with regard to questions about how to live. The idea of neutrality suggests the spurious conception of 'objectivity' discussed in connection with the 'fact–value' gap in Chapter 2: it implies that the tutor can meaningfully be said to assume a 'value-neutral' perspective and that any evaluative stance taken up by the students is in contrast 'merely' their own subjective opinion. It suggests, implicitly, that there is a 'privileged' perspective on moral matters, but it avoids the accusation of moral dogmatism by making that perspective an empty one: the position of 'neutrality'. The dogma this in fact communicates is that the truly impartial person is the person who has no substantial view on matters of right and wrong, such that to have any view at all, however sensible and well thought out, is to be 'partial'. If the tutor were to intervene in order to condemn a particular student's comments for being (for example) homophobic, then he could be condemned for being 'biased'. No matter how clear his arguments were and however good a demonstration of moral reasoning his interjection provided, the students could complain that he was 'using his position' to convey his own 'personal opinion'. In short, the structure of the discussion implicitly conveys a philosophical picture which may have been in influence (perhaps not consciously) when the approach was designed and this picture is in line with the various forms of ethical subjectivism presented and criticised in Chapters 2 and 5.[6]

It is no surprise, then, that this approach has come under pressure, both from theorists and from those involved with the formation of education policy. If reasoning is to have any goal then this goal must be some conclusion. If no conclusion is really any better than any other then what, precisely, is the point of reasoning? The postmodernists considered in Chapter 2 at least understood this: if the object of rational thought is the truth and there is no truth to be discovered (or if the truth is a merely 'personal truth' about one's own private prejudices) then rational thought must be abandoned. All that can remain is rhetoric: the attempt to use persuasive language to convince others to take up the stances to which one is (for no good reason) personally committed. So such discussions are likely to produce not critical reasoning skills but rather the skills of the political hack: to sway others around to one's favoured opinion by the use of persuasive language.

On the other hand, if reasoning does have a goal then that goal (it might be argued), in the field of moral education, must be the communication of the right values to the students. In which case, we must be able to identify those values and if we can do so then why choose so uncertain (and philosophically problematic) a method of conveying them to students as a discussion wherein the teacher must remain 'neutral'? This brings us to the second approach, which Wringe (1998b, p. 280) characterises as 'inculcatory . . . in which prescriptions are enunciated and assertively enforced'. The thinking behind this approach seems to be that 'neutrality' in moral matters is neither possible nor desirable. Instead we should be looking for effective ways to 'transmit' the values and associated modes of behaviour which we regard as central to our way of life (ibid, p. 279).

Clearly this (characteristically conservative) approach is regaining popularity, both among sections of the populace who (somewhat simplistically) view the (characteristically liberal) approach based on debate as responsible for the decline of 'discipline' in schools and also with such influential groups as the Schools Curriculum and Assessment Authority (SCAA). Wringe cites a document produced by the SCAA in 1996 which sets out a range of 'value statements' followed by a series of prescriptions prefaced by the words 'On the basis of these values we should . . .'. The Chief Executive of the SCAA described the document as 'a statement of what we as a society are authorising schools to transmit on our behalf' – values which (if need be) can be 'inculcated in a straightforwardly didactic way' (ibid, p. 280).

Wringe is rightly sceptical about the potential effectiveness of this approach. Values are not 'high level moral prescriptions' from which one deduces specific commands (ibid, p. 281). You do not affect a person's values simply by telling her in very general terms what is right and wrong. Rather, to talk of a person's values is to talk about what motivates that person. It is to discuss what types of concern strike her as relevant in determining the conduct of her life: to value certain things is to be disposed to act in certain ways. In a society which overtly promotes crude materialistic egoism, where people freeze to death in the streets and where vast numbers of citizens are condemned to a lifetime of unfulfilling, mechanistic labour, the attempt to lecture students 'didactically' about the values of unselfishness, respect for 'human rights' and the 'uniqueness' of each human being will strike any reasonably intelligent student as rank hypocrisy.[7] In the absence of any reasoned arguments in support of specific value judgements, without any clear account of why certain ways of living are supposed to be preferable to others, this brand of 'education' is likely to breed only deep (and entirely justified) cynicism. Wringe notes that the SCAA document studiously avoids the use of the word 'therefore' in linking its general 'value statements' to specific prescriptions, employing instead the phrase: 'On the basis of these values we should . . .'. This is a 'dishonest device' which suggests the same sense as 'therefore' while 'evading the critical scrutiny use of this word invites'. He raises two crucial questions concerning this whole approach:

> *'1. Why should we give our moral approval to traits of character and modes of behaviour just because they support a particular way of life?*
>
> *2. Supposing we could justify so doing, how are we to characterise our own society and its way of life as a preliminary to identifying the most important virtues its citizens need to develop and the proper manner of their exercise?' (Wringe 1998a, p. 228)*

To take the second question first, it strikes me that the Chief

Executive of the SCAA displays the characteristic arrogance of a person being paid far too much for what he does, in claiming the document produced by his organisation somehow speaks for 'society' as a whole. Distressing as it may be to philosophical conservatives, there is very little in the way of 'consensus' upon important moral questions in contemporary society. (This is presumably why the 'value statements' are kept so vague and general and their logical links with specific prescriptions are left unclear.) If we are to expect people to accept some specific set of value judgements, with concrete implications for how they should live their lives, then we surely owe them some sort of explanation, other than appeal to the 'authority of consensus' (Wringe 1998b, p. 279) which is in any case spurious. This brings us to the first question. Without the element of critical reflection and argument, there is no discernible difference between this brand of 'education' and simple 'indoctrination'. So defenders of this approach must either supplement their position with rational arguments in favour of the 'values' they presume to 'transmit' (reintroducing the notion of 'moral reasoning') or they must be prepared to deny (however implausibly) the intelligibility of Wringe's question.

Given the philosophical underpinnings of their position, some defenders of this view would seem prepared to take the latter option. Wringe notes a certain irony in that its defenders make it a key virtue of this approach that it combats 'relativism', while justifying it intellectually with reference to assumptions that any philosopher would recognise as patently relativistic. That is to say, the only argument it is thought necessary to offer for the choice of values to be 'inculcated' is that these values are 'ours' (ibid, p. 282) – they represent and reinforce types of behaviour which help to sustain ways of life of which 'we' approve. The question of why we *should* approve of these ways of life (and so, crucially, why we should expect anyone else to) is treated as somehow not arising.

Conventionalism

To avoid confusion it might be useful to distinguish the form of 'relativism' defenders of this approach dislike from the form they typically presuppose. What they object to is a range of different positions on questions of value being open to students (and citizens generally) such that each individual may choose any one she pleases, there being no grounds (other than purely subjective preference) to judge any one superior to any other. In short they object to what I have described (Chapter 5) as 'subjectivism' or 'irrationalism', usually because they fear it as a threat to social cohesion. The form of relativism they pre-suppose can be labelled 'conventionalism', the view that questions of value can be decisively settled by reference to agreements between groups of people. Such agreements are neither explicit nor rational (unlike the contract myth described in Chapter 6) but rather they are non-rational and (typically) implicit,[8] and they define what 'rationality' means within a given context. Social practices simply 'evolve' and 'give rise' to values. Knowing how to live is, on this view, a matter of knowing the conventions which govern the practices in which one is engaged. So to teach someone how to live is to instil in her a set of values – to generate attitudes and consequent habits of behaviour that accord with the conventions of the practices which characterise a given 'way of life'. The norms which define that way of life determine what is right or wrong for anyone living within the community whose 'way' it is, so Wringe's question (why should we approve of something just because it supports a given way of life?) becomes unintelligible. The answer that something is 'what we do around here' becomes the end of the line as far as moral explanations go.

I have argued against this view (and some slightly more interesting forms of relativism) elsewhere (Loughlin and Pritchard 1997, 1998). Conventionalism is little more than a mutation of irrationalism proper (Loughlin 1998a, pp. 23 and 30). It is in essence a crude response to the fact–value gap. Noting that what we have reason to do is controversial and cannot in any straightforward or logically valid way be read off 'the facts', the conventionalist (like the emotivist considered in Chapter 5) assumes that the faculty of human reasoning cannot guide us in the conduct of our lives. Instead of concluding that we may therefore believe anything we like about evaluative questions (the conclusion which would in fact follow if the assumption were correct) the conventionalist, fearing (for reasons already suggested) the subjectivism this conclusion would imply, searches for an alternative and notes that we can still talk about which values are 'correct' so long as we mean 'correct according to the conventions which operate in this or that community'. While the identity conditions of a 'community' are inherently unclear (for most conventionalists it appears to be a social entity somewhat larger than a single family but is not necessarily anything so large as an entire nation) if we accept this constraint upon our critical faculties it becomes possible to determine what is right and wrong in a 'rational' way: by finding out what people in fact think about such questions in the communities of which we are a part.

While the honest irrationalism of the logical positivists has fallen out of fashion in academic circles, conventionalism still commands substantial support. It provides a useful theoretical apology for just about any unreflective moral stance. Whether I am a fox-hunter, a religious fanatic who wants to beat his wife and have his daughter circumcised or an Ulster loyalist determined to intimidate and taunt his neighbours by marching past their homes displaying all the symbols of their historical subservience – I have an automatic defence by appeal to the 'values' of 'my community'. (Furthermore, there will be academics prepared to champion my cause, from the political left or the political right – depending largely on my race and social class.) If you point out that I have no arguments in support of the substantial moral claims I make I can, just like the logical positivist, look at you incredulously and ask you what on earth you mean. However, unlike the positivist, I am not thereby obliged to admit that my stance has no rational basis: indeed, so long as I can identify a group of people who agree with me, I can claim that my stance is very rational – for a person of my sort. Learn this one theoretical argument and you will never have to defend anything you believe ever again.

Some form of this doctrine appears to be at work in Dracopoulou's defence (1998) of her fellow bioethicists against my arguments expressed in Chapter 6. Responding to my claims that such theorists treat the context which gives rise to the problems they discuss as morally unproblematic, thereby providing an apology for the brutality and injustice of the rationing process, Dracopoulou concludes that I am committed to the belief in 'an all-embracing rationality' which presupposes 'a notion of morality which is abstract, ahistorical and static' (ibid, pp. 9–10). But this is wrong because really morality:

> '*is an institution of life that is constantly evolving, as part of continually changing social circumstances and cultural and historical traditions. A context-free morality in which reason and justification are a matter of deducing certain moral judgements and certain ethical codes from pre-existing universal principles is inconsistent with the realistic conception of morality as a complex institution which is inseparable from a matrix of beliefs and attitudes of particular cultures at particular times in history.*' (ibid, p. 10)

Dracopoulou concludes that managers can engage in 'contextual moral reasoning' which 'is stronger' than the 'ahistorical' kind because it 'allows for the richness and complexities of situations to be captured and thus avoids oversimplification'.

It is not immediately obvious what any of this has to do with my arguments. If Dracopoulou thinks I am defending a view of moral reasoning based on an infallible awareness of abstract principles, from which one 'deduces' 'ethical codes', or if she thinks my view is that to think rationally one needs to be blind to the 'richness and complexities' of specific situations, then just like Wall (whose 'general approach' (op cit) as someone on 'the other side of the debate' from me she claims to 'support'), she 'replies' to a position that is quite the reverse of my own. The points she cites against me are central components of my critique of the bioethics she is defending. I have argued that, while bioethicists can talk all they like about the 'values', 'goals' or 'principles' which in their view should 'inform' or in some sense be the 'basis for' practice, what they say lacks even the potential to influence practice in any meaningful way because what individuals do in the specific contexts where decisions actually take place is likely to be influenced by features of those contexts which are unique. This is (one of the reasons) why we have to rethink the role of theory in practical decision making, if theory is to have any role at all in influencing practice. Unless we take account of the genuine conceptual difficulties in the process of 'applying' theory to practice, we risk reinforcing simplistic pictures of the nature of theorising and of social reality. In that case the only practical consequence of our work will be to foster an entirely illusory sense that what happens in practice is 'based on' rational thought and is therefore more 'ethical' than it would otherwise be. The political consequences of this situation were spelled out in some detail in Chapter 6 and in the article to which Dracopoulou is replying (Loughlin 1998b).

I do not, however, think that Dracopoulou has simply (and certainly not completely) misunderstood my position. She has identified a feature of my approach to moral reasoning to which she (sincerely, and wrongly) objects. To see what this is it is useful to consider her support for my rejection of 'irrationalism'. She states:

> 'Emotivism, like the position of the logical positivists from which it derives, has long been discredited.' (Dracopoulou 1998, p. 9)

However, she also states that we do not need to appeal to so 'extreme' a view to reject my position on the nature of moral thinking. Clearly, she sees her own view about rationality and morality as in some way a compromise between two extremes: on the one hand my belief in an 'all-embracing' rationality, which allows that even social contexts and conventions are subject to rational criticism, and the irrationalist view on the other hand, which reduces reason to the discovery of the best means to achieve one's arbitrary (non-rational) ends (whatever they happen to be). The talk of morality as an 'evolving institution' (rather than a method of critical thinking) which is 'inseparable' from a 'matrix' of the beliefs of particular 'cultures' (as opposed to the thinking of particular human beings) suggests the conventionalism sketched above.

This reading has the virtue of making sense of Dracopoulou's response: it would explain what is supposed to be wrong with my arguments. I claimed that the context which gives rise to certain social roles must itself be subject to philosophical scrutiny: its moral status cannot be taken as read and individuals working within specific social roles may find that it is some feature of that context which stands in the way of their finding morally adequate solutions to the problems they encounter. But if conventionalism is right then it is not clear what it means to criticise a social context, since the meaning of 'morally adequate solutions' can only be understood with reference to the 'matrix of beliefs and attitudes' which define that context.

Hence Dracopoulou is incredulous of my claim that the 'key virtue' of philosophical methods of reasoning is that they enable individuals to think 'beyond their roles' (ibid, p. 7), a view which she sees as 'opposite to' the view that 'rationality is practical' (ibid, p. 9). On the account of moral thinking to which she seems committed, properly 'practical' reasoning is:

> *'essentially continuous with the case-driven, induc-tive process of seeking a solution to a problem, carried out within a framework of central cultural values and guiding norms . . .' (ibid, p. 10. Dracopoulou is citing Winkler here but with total approval)*

These 'norms' include 'professional functions'. It becomes hard (if not impossible) to see what it might mean to criticise these 'norms' of practice since they provide the 'framework' of 'values' within which all rational thinking takes place. To be a 'rational' person is (by definition) to be 'guided' by these norms.

It is worth noting that this is not quite so different from the 'extreme' views of people like Ayer, which I discussed in Chapter 5, as Dracopoulou apparently thinks. For Ayer (as we saw), the role of philosophy was to solve problems (largely through the clarification of the meanings of key terms) which arise within specific contexts, not to discover moral truths which could provide the basis for a rational criticism of these contexts. Given the arbitrary commitment to a particular set of values, the logical positivist can happily agree that we can 'justify' some specific moral imperatives – conditionally, mean-ing, on the assumption of those values. This is just a develop-ment of the concept of 'means–end' rationality: if you want to live a certain sort of life, then it is rational to do some things and not others. If I want to avoid violence, then it is rational for me to avoid certain forms of behaviour and so to avoid cultivating those feelings or dispositions (for instance, the propensity to react aggressively when insulted) which might lead me to engage in such behaviour. On the other hand, if I have chosen to adopt a violent lifestyle, then it is 'rational' for me to cultivate different dispositions: we might say (for instance) that in that case I ought not to be upset by the sight of my fellow human beings in great pain. Both the positivist and the conventionalist agree that it is not possible to answer the question as to why I should adopt certain ways of living in the first place. To ask the question is (they think) to commit a philosophical error.

They differ, however, over the precise nature of that error. For the positivist the error is the assumption that it is possible to give a rational answer to any genuinely evaluative question: questions about how we should live are (on this view) purely matters of personal preference. For the conventionalist, the error is in failing to see that 'ways of living' provide the standard for judgements about rationality, such that a person who does not see why he should adopt the values of his community is (by definition) someone who has failed to 'learn the difference between right and wrong'. Why this should follow is by no means clear. If 'this is my way' does not constitute a rational argument (which clearly it doesn't) it is, to say the least, not obvious why 'this is our way' should do so. As a matter of empirical fact, people do develop their personal moral stances within social contexts and so they will often come to adopt the values of the people around them, but this is in no sense an argument to the effect that they *should* do so.

To a consistent irrationalist like Ayer, if an individual finds himself living amongst people whose values he does not share, there is no philosophically significant sense in which he can be judged 'wrong'. One might argue that, judged against the 'framework' of their values, he is 'wrong' but one might equally point out that judged against the framework of his values, they are 'wrong'. In the absence of any further arguments (about the relative merits of each 'framework') the debate can go no further. The claim that he is part of their community, therefore he ought to adopt their values, would seem to fall foul of the 'fact–value' gap in a particularly clumsy manner. If membership of a given community is to be equated with certain duties or morally binding commitments, then it is not a simple 'matter of fact' – it is not (for instance) a matter of living within a particular geographical area. Rather, it is contingent upon accepting the values of the community in the first place, so to the extent that I reject the values of 'my' community it may be incorrect to describe it as 'my community'. As Wringe (1998b, pp. 282–3) puts it:

> 'To speak of a group's values may be to imply that the holding of those values is definitive of membership of the group in question. Not to be committed or to conform to those values is simply not to belong to the group, to be an outsider . . .'

He makes the astute point that the problem with the word 'values' is not, as some authors have claimed, that the term itself 'automatically implies notions of vagueness or relativism, but that it is characteristically used descriptively' (ibid, p. 282). Descriptively, we may speak of 'the macho values of a group of young males', the 'peaceable values of a Quaker community', 'the aristocratic values of the Prussian officer class' (op cit) or indeed the values of any social group or single individual. In doing so we do not commit ourselves to approving or disapproving of any particular set of values, so we do not say anything which requires defence in terms of rational moral arguments. In other words, although we talk *about* values, we do not make any genuinely *evaluative* claims.

To say that certain people believe that this or that is right or wrong is not to make any claims about what *is* right or wrong which would invite the questions: 'why do you think that?' and 'why should anyone else agree with you?' To answer these questions one would have to do more than simply point out that certain other people do in fact think the same way. Instead, one would need to provide good reasons to favour certain types of behaviour over others.

This brings out the key error which the conventionalist approach to moral thinking embodies. Via the use of the word 'values', properly evaluative questions can easily be translated into descriptive questions. So in answering the question: 'what has value?' (meaning: what sort of thing do we have good reason to value?) or: 'what types of behaviour are valuable to society?' (meaning: what forms of conduct, if generally adopted, would actually serve to make our society a better one?) it is easy to slip into talk of 'what the values are' of persons or social groups of certain sorts. But statements of this latter type are really descriptions, not value judgements: they tell us what certain people think about what is valuable, how they in fact conduct their business. As we have seen (Chapter 2, under the heading 'Facts and values'), the knowledge that people do behave in certain ways or approve of certain things does not provide us with the answer to the bona fide evaluative question: 'should we also behave in those ways or approve of those things?' The conventionalist commits a version of what has been called the 'descriptive fallacy' (Hare 1983, pp. 111–26, 1972, pp. 24–9) by treating claims about what particular groups of people in fact do (at a given time and/or in a given place) as somehow settling the issue as to what they should do.

To grasp fully the intellectual poverty of this approach to moral reasoning it is probably sufficient to consider just one practical example. When a doctor and prominent advocate of active euthanasia[9] was put on trial in the United States for giving a lethal injection to a terminally ill patient (at the patient's request) many of the arguments levelled against him reflected the influence of conventionalism. Several commentators objected that it was not the commonly understood 'role' of the doctor to kill his patients, however much pain they were in and however much they wanted to die. To act in this way was to misunderstand the 'values' that 'underpin' medical practice. By 'medical doctor' we mean (amongst other things) 'someone dedicated to saving life', not someone prepared to terminate life.

Now suppose we accept this. Suppose we agree that this person acted in a way contrary to generally understood conventions about what it is to be a medical doctor. Does it follow that he acted wrongly? My previous points about membership of a community bring out a very obvious response. He could simply refuse to accept the conventional characterisation of the doctor's role, arguing instead that he was part of a different practice, and according to the conventions of that practice, it is sometimes legitimate to kill your patients: for instance, if they are terminally ill, in great pain and have competently requested death. (And, obviously, so long as one does so in a way that is painless and respectful to the dying patient.) To be engaged in this distinct form of medical practice, it is necessary (let us say) to accept many of the values of traditional medicine, but not to accept those specific values with regard to the so-called 'sanctity of life' as understood by the opponents of active euthanasia. He would not even have to give up calling himself a 'medical doctor' to give this response, since it is not clear that members of any particular practice have exclusive right to a given label. The conventionalist, of all people, should accept that no one sect amongst the Christians has exclusive ownership of the term 'Christian', so why should only one group amongst medical doctors (be it the pro- or anti-euthanasia camp) have sole claim to being the 'true' medics?

This response is particularly effective when one considers that the identity conditions of a given 'community' or 'practice' are left quite deliberately (and necessarily) vague by the conventionalist. As Dracopoulou cheerfully points out, the 'cultural and historical traditions' which supposedly provide the 'frameworks' for moral thinking are 'constantly evolving' and so are 'continually changing'. It follows that members of the pro-euthanasia camp could argue that their practice was simply another stage in the 'evolution' of traditional medical practice. However, it would also seem that their opponents could, with equal legitimacy, insist that the 'tradition' of medical practice was clearly opposed to euthanasia. Without any basis for rational criticism of the alternative practices or frameworks, one must simply choose (on non-rational grounds) between them, so conventionalism collapses into the honest subjectivism from which it emerged.

Even if we assume it is possible to assess in some definitive way what a given 'tradition' thinks about any specific issue, clearly one does not do so by employing *philosophical* methods of inquiry, so the idea that this line of thinking can deflect criticisms of 'applied ethics' is a non-starter.[10] A serious investigation of the 'values' of a community or professional group would surely be a *sociological* inquiry. One would need to find out (through empirical research) what people within a given culture, at a given point in time, actually thought about specific questions, how members of the group under investigation typically responded to certain problems and so forth. Such an inquiry would not be helped by philosophical speculation on what their values 'should be'. Depending on how fast the culture is 'evolving', the information gathered may soon be out of date and it is in any case (for the reasons given) not clear why the conclusions of such a study would provide a 'guide' to anyone on how to live and practise. It could at most tell them what to do if they wanted to fit in with members of the group, but it is (logically) incapable of justifying the (evaluative) premise that they should want to 'fit in'.

Moral realism

So the only consistent alternative to irrationalism is moral realism, the view that it is possible for human subjects to stand back from the practices, conventions and contexts which shape their professional and social roles and to subject those practices and contexts to rational criticism, by considering what reasons one might have for approving of some ways of living as opposed to others. It is because she recognises the moral realism implicit in my criticisms of bioethics that Dracopoulou ascribes to me a view of rationality as 'all-embracing'. We are not, on this view, limited to reasoning within a set of assumptions about what is acceptable, that are 'given' by the practices in which we happen to be involved. We do not engage our rational faculties, simply nor even primarily, in our capacities as representatives of particular social or professional groups, but as *human beings*, blessed with brains and hearts and with the duty to engage them if we are to live anything that can plausibly be called a full human life. Rationality applies to the conduct of a life *as such*: in principle I can think about anything I do and question whether or not I should be doing it, or doing it in a particular way. Therefore moral reasoning is not (or is not just) a matter of discovering the 'values' which underlie our practices, since once we have done this we can think about whether we should approve of those values. To such a thinker 'this is just what people of our sort do' is never a convincing answer, since what one wants to know is why one should be that sort of person in the first place.

What is supposed to be wrong with this account of moral reasoning and the broad conception of moral life which it supports? Dracopoulou rejects this account because, she claims, it makes morality 'abstract, ahistorical and static'. It is important to think carefully about what this claim is supposed to mean and why it functions as an objection to my view. With respect to Dracopoulou, who strikes me as a decent and intelligent sort of person, the style of argument (and interestingly also the writing style[11]) at this point in her discussion is reminiscent of a style discussed in Chapter 2, in connection with postmodernist critiques of 'reason' and 'truth'. Take a perfectly straightforward claim. Translate it into a bizarre-sounding metaphysical claim, then assume an attitude of incredulity towards it. (This, I gather, is what it is to 'problematize' a claim.) Then, with little or no analysis of the position suitably 'problematized', present your own favoured position (preferably with very little explanation of what it in fact entails) as if it were the only credible alternative and close the discussion.

In Chapter 2, the claim in question was that it is possible to think rationally about how one ought to live. That was translated into the claim that one has achieved a 'transcendent' perspective, which was promptly declared impossible. In this case the claim is that it is possible to evaluate social contexts, as well as the actions of individuals within those contexts, and that there are times when it is reasonable to conclude that the reason why a person can't find an adequate solution is not because she hasn't tried hard enough: rather it is because of the constraints imposed by the context. In such cases, we must work to change the context, since working within it we can only find inadequate solutions. In the meantime we must be honest about the situation, avoiding the pretence that the context is compatible with finding adequate solutions, since this is the way to ensure that the context will never change.

These claims are accordingly translated into the claim about abstract, ahistorical and static moral truths. Put like this it sounds suddenly rather confusing. If all this claim means is that we can reasonably judge some social contexts to be better than others, then I am committed to this view – and so is anyone with a heart and a brain free of corruption. In medieval societies they used to burn people as witches and in contemporary capitalist societies they don't. In this respect, contemporary capitalist societies are an improvement on medieval societies, because they are free of this particular form of barbarity. In contrast, medieval societies did not pollute the world to such an extent as to threaten a major ecological catastrophe. In this respect contemporary capitalist societies compare unfavourably with their predecessors. If the belief in an 'ahistorical' morality means simply that this sort of comparison is rationally possible, then what sane person could sincerely dispute it? If it means anything else, then Dracopoulou should really say what else it means and she should explain why exactly she thinks I am committed to it. Wringe puts it well:

> 'Communities are not hermetically sealed units of incommensurable value systems but may themselves be criticised on moral grounds, both from within and from without. We have no difficulty in approving of outstanding individuals who have been critical of their own communities and, in some cases, have paid for it with their lives. We are equally unhesitating in our criticisms of societies with their own internal constellations of virtues and values which seem plainly evil or perverse. The aristocratic code of honour that led a seventeenth century French nobleman to run his tailor through with his sword for presenting his bill, or the set of values that more recently led to the extermination of whole trainloads of victims deemed decadent are example enough.' (Wringe 1998a, p. 229)

Our ability to criticise the conventions underlying whole ways of life is as fundamental to our common-sense conception of moral thinking as our ability to identify physical objects is to our understanding of who we are and our relationship with the external world. It strikes me that there is a fundamental question of philosophical methodology at stake here. If a theory causes us to be sceptical about the most obvious features of rational life, does that give us grounds to deny those features of rational life or to search for a better theory – one that is able to make sense of them?

Given my earlier points about the nature and justification of the activity of theorising (Chapters 1 and 5), we should give the latter answer. We are not required to 'work within' the conceptualisations of our lives and practices which are 'supplied' by the 'context' in which we find ourselves. It is definitive of our status as human subjects that we can subject those very conceptualisations, and the practices which give rise to them, to critical scrutiny. If I come to the conclusion that the way in which people within my own society do business is fundamentally flawed, because the 'framework of cultural values' we have inherited is in many important respects perverse, this does not necessarily show that my parents and teachers have failed me with regard to my moral education – that I have been 'badly brought up'. Indeed, it may show quite the reverse. It is only because people can distance themselves in this way from the 'values' of the dominant social order and its 'institutions' and 'traditions' that genuine social progress (as opposed, merely, to social change) is even a logical possibility.

As theorists we need to make sense of this phenomenon, by developing a coherent account of the rational processes which make it possible to discover the flaws inherent within a way of life – even from one's perspective 'within' it. Rather than attempting so serious a theoretical task, it may seem easier to take up a theoretical stance which declares any such account impossible: just as it is in some ways easier to be sceptical about the existence of the independent world than to develop a coherent account of our knowledge of it. What is not so easy is to take up such a stance while claiming sincerely that one has anything worthwhile to say. By denying the possibility of 'criteria of appraisal external to particular societies' (Wringe, op cit) conventionalism makes it impossible to give an intuitively sound account of one of the most basic features of moral existence and so it stands alongside the vat–brain theory (Chapter 1) as another thesis unfit for employment within the context of a rational life.

If we can criticise the values of entire social orders then we can certainly criticise the values which shape and delimit specific professional roles within those social orders. There is nothing mysterious about the claim that a context can leave no morally adequate solutions open: an obvious example would be the sort of case concerning health services organisation discussed in Chapter 6, where the context of scarcity and the associated value of economic efficiency require me to choose between two courses of action, both of which condemn some of my fellow human beings to suffering and death. This seems plainly to be an empirical possibility and we do not help individuals work out how to respond to such situations by constructing bogus 'solutions' which rationalise the barbarity of such a choice.

The meaning of 'morally adequate' here is something like: 'decent – fair and humane', and I would suggest that our understanding of these concepts derives from our common humanity. Of course we learn their meaning within social contexts, in the sense that I develop my intuitions about how to treat my fellows by actually coming across them. (Thus, there is a perfectly legitimate sense in which I may not know what it means to do well in a specific context without practical experience of that very context and the real persons who populate it.) It obviously does not follow from this that the conventions of the context are beyond moral criticism or that they should have the final word on how I do treat my fellows. If it did then debates about moral education would be utterly meaningless, since any context at all, however alienating and brutalising, would provide an 'education' in some set of 'values', encouraging certain character traits and intuitive responses within the subjects exposed to that context. We can debate moral education (and ethics more generally) because we know that contexts which encourage deceitfulness, mistrust of and callousness towards one's fellows are poor contexts, ones which repress our best human capacities and so stifle proper human flourishing.

Furthermore, if we are prepared to call any context characterised by shared social practices a 'community' then we do violence to this concept. I find it disturbing that, in discussions of 'applied ethics', the label 'communitarianism' is increasingly being used to signify the doctrine I have discussed under the label 'conventionalism'. For instance, Chadwick (1998, p. 63) describes the 'community approach' to ethics in health management as based on the idea that 'values are derived from practices and ways of living', such that the ethical manager should 'try to determine what the values of the community are – to elucidate a communitarian consensus'. Yet clearly some contexts provide a better basis for the development of decent attitudes, and a proper sense of community, than others.

Consider a group of people whose 'consensus' is that some sections of the population may be subject to systematic violence at the hands of others and that the victims ought to accept this for the sake of the 'community', whose stability and very identity depend upon the perpetuation of its traditional practices.[12] If these people are to be called 'communitarians', then we need to find some other label for those who think the concept of 'community' has more substantial moral content than this: or else this view will pass quietly out of the picture, having been defined away in the unhelpful debate between 'communitarians' and 'individualists'. If there are no constraints on how a 'moral community' may treat the individuals that make it up, then any gathering of ruffians can be such a community. There is no obvious reason why, given so weak a definition of community, the most brutal individualist social order should not qualify, so long as its members are committed to the shared values of competition and the 'winner take all' ethos. A more meaningful notion of 'community' would have to specify standards of decency to which any group's collective behaviour must conform before the group can count as a 'community'. Thus to make sense of a worthwhile concept of 'community' we need to be moral realists – we must believe it is possible to evaluate communal practices and social contexts in terms of some more general conception of human decency.

Living well: individuality, community and the meaning of life

What follows from all this – for moral education generally and for the specific project of this book: to determine what, if anything, a work of theory may helpfully say to individuals sincerely concerned to improve their thinking about practical matters in the area of health services organisation (and indeed in other areas of professional and social life)? One conclusion to be drawn from the immediately preceding comments is that there is no very clear-cut distinction between questions of political philosophy and questions of moral education. Both concern the nature of a decent social environment and the sort of attitudes that such an environment should foster. We learn how to live within specific environments and so the nature of the social environment will inevitably be an important factor in determining the sort of people we become. Wringe (1998b, p. 284) makes a similar point, noting that moral education is 'a social process' whose goal is to affect behaviour by affecting people's characters, not 'to increase the occurrences of pious utterances in the world'. It follows that: 'we cannot successfully teach one value when our institutions demonstrate that we are committed to others'. He goes on (ibid, pp. 285–6) to develop implications about the nature of the school environment. There are, I think, some pertinent implications for the educational and working environments of managers in the health service, and the role of management organisations in fostering these environments, which it will be necessary to consider shortly.

I noted above that Wringe seems concerned to combine the two approaches to moral education sketched in this chapter in a way that avoids their respective pitfalls but preserves their advantages, and that he does this by appealing to the Aristotelian idea of moral life as the development and exercise of the 'virtues': those traits of character which enable a person to live a fulfilling human life (to 'flourish'). It seems to me that there are a couple of other (related) philosophical projects underway in the articles I have cited. One is to affect some kind of reconciliation between approaches to ethics which take the concept of 'autonomy' (which Wringe labels 'self-direction') as fundamental to understanding the nature of moral life and those which view the point of ethics as promoting the 'good life'. The other is to demonstrate that there is no necessary opposition between 'living rightly' and 'living well': between doing one's duties to others and living as good a life as one possibly can. Indeed, properly understood, one cannot live well unless one also lives rightly.

As we have seen, defenders of the 'inculcatory' approach to moral education were right to reject the idea of 'neutrality' at work in the approach based on 'moral reasoning': the very activity of encouraging discussion presupposes that a discussion of the type encouraged is valuable, so this is not a morally neutral approach. Values concern the way we live our lives: to value some things is to believe that one has reason to choose certain courses of action over others, to adopt some habits of thought and behaviour and not others. In everything we say and do, some assumptions about what is valuable are at work. This is particularly evident in the way we think it appropriate to treat others, especially if we are engaged in something we consider to be an 'educative' project. By its very social nature, education cannot be neutral between competing moral stances.

Therefore, defenders of the 'inculcatory' approach are also correct in asserting that we are unavoidably engaged in communicating values when we attempt to educate, so we need to make decisions about the sort of character traits we want to encourage. The attempt to deny that we are contributing to the shaping of a person's character, and so to avoid questions about the sort of contribution we want to make, does not mean that our treatment of them will have no effect. It is more likely to mean that our treatment will have effects we do not intend, such as fostering a sense that moral thinking is a frivolous or subjective matter. Since we are unavoidably in the business of fostering certain traits of character, Wringe concludes that we should attempt to foster those character traits that will enable a person to live well: to promote virtuous characters. As noted at various places in this text, the point of education must be to produce the right sort of people to face the world. The question of course arises as to how one determines who is the 'right sort' of person.

What is outrageous about the views of many defenders of this approach is that they see no need for any justification for the values they attempt to instil in their students, other than the claim that these values support 'our' way of life. As a matter of sociological fact, it is very difficult, in the context of a pluralistic society, to say anything terribly precise about what 'our' values are: people are presented with a range of different, apparently credible positions on a number of moral questions. We must find some rational way to defend some values over others, for any sensible student will recognise and resist the arbitrary imposition of a set of values as an attempt to indoctrinate her into a given way of life. The concept of moral reasoning cannot be abandoned, since in a very obvious way, the attempt to ignore or repress the development of students' critical and analytical faculties is the attempt to discourage a key human virtue. Insofar as there are any value judgements that are shared by the vast majority of reasonably sane persons, the unreflective, dogmatic, unintelligent human being is obviously not 'our' model of human success. Indeed, the very project of defending a way of life based on these character traits would be profoundly paradoxical, if not straightforwardly contradictory, since anyone sufficiently intelligent to want to listen attentively to the defence would already be committed to rejecting the way of life defended. The person who mindlessly follows rules, who never attempts to understand his world or the problems which confront him, who decides how to live on the basis of what he thinks others will approve of, who sees no need to justify any of the claims he makes or to inquire into the basis of his own beliefs – in short, someone who never feels the need to think for himself – could not plausibly be said to be living a full human life and yet this is the very sort of person most likely to be successfully 'educated' by the inculcatory approach. (In contrast, the independent thinker is more likely to be viewed as a 'problem student' by practitioners of this approach.)

This helps to clarify what we do mean by the 'right sort' of person and to provide a defensible conception of moral education, one which combines what is good in each approach. Far from remaining neutral about what is good in life, we must promote, unapologetically, the virtue of critical thinking and all that this entails. We must defend the values of intellectual honesty, rigour and integrity and bring out clearly their links with such central values as human freedom. The attentive reader will notice that this is what I have been doing throughout this text. By inviting her to join me in rigorous intellectual exercise concerning what matters most in life, I have attempted to encourage a certain style of thinking which I have identified as an essential form of 'intellectual and moral self-defence' against the corrupting influences of the modern world. I have noted that unless we are able to question our own fundamental assumptions, to think creatively about the pictures of our lives and practices which influence our behaviour and to remain open to the possibility that what we have so far taken for granted is wrong, the way we think and consequently the way we live will be determined by forces we do not understand, let alone control. Thus our lives will not, in any meaningful sense, be our own. Wringe expresses a similar idea when he argues that:

'Moral independence, owning and taking possession of one's life, may be seen as a kind of master-virtue . . . '
(Wringe 1998a, p. 235)

The distinction between teaching 'reasoning skills' and 'communicating values' is misleading, since to reason well is to develop one's intellectual and moral instincts, which is to develop the virtues of self-direction and critical thinking. Rational life is a sort of practice: far from being morally neutral, the activity of critical thinking constitutes a *way of life,* embodying the commitment to employ one's definitive human capacities in the search for the truth about matters of value and indeed about all aspects of one's condition. The day I stop questioning (both my own preconceptions and the 'official line' on any issue) is the day I relinquish membership of the community of rational beings: a group that the dogmatists and slogan-mongers in government and business seem determined to drive to extinction. The day that I cease to take care in the process of forming my beliefs and attitudes is, in truth, the day that *I* cease to form them at all. From that day onwards I will be swept along by whatever cultural tide assaults me: prod me and I move this way or that, but never under my own steam.

This goes some of the way to breaking down the dichotomy between approaches to ethics based on autonomy and those based on living well. It makes little sense to say that someone's life has gone well if that person has no control over her own destiny, if her personal development is a matter of what I described above as a form of psychological inertia. Wringe (ibid, p. 234) describes a range of 'good lives' corresponding to various ways in which people may find meaning and fulfilment. One might take an interest in art, music or political ideals; or one might devote oneself to caring for non-human animals or to protecting the natural environment;[13] or one might simply take joy in developing friendships with the people one happens to encounter. All of these forms of good living are possible within the framework of 'self-direction', although tellingly they all involve taking an interest in something outside oneself.

This brings us to the relationship between 'living rightly' (fulfilling one's obligations towards others) and 'living well'. To say that the good life requires self-determination is not to say it involves being inward looking or selfish. To learn how to live well is not to learn how to satisfy one's arbitrary whims. It is to think about the sort of dispositions one wants to develop, which is in turn to think about the sort of relationships with one's fellows that one must develop if one is to live a decent human life. For Aristotle, a virtue always had two corresponding vices, being the rational 'mean' between possible excesses. (It is via this idea that the concept of 'balance' enters our moral vocabulary: so to treat others in a fair and decent manner is to be 'well balanced', while a person who behaves unreasonably will sometimes be thought of as 'unbalanced'.) Thus when Wringe suggests that a key virtue we need to develop in the modern world is 'self-assertiveness' (ibid, p. 235) he does not mean what (one imagines) many senior managers and politicians understand by this term. He means that we do not live well if we are overly dependent upon or dominated by or exploited by others, but nor do we live well if we are the ones who dominate, exploit or override the interests of others. To live life engaged in the project of controlling others is just as bad for oneself as it is to live under the arbitrary control of another, since in each case one falls short of living what can meaningfully be considered a 'good' human life.

It strikes me that the egoist considered in Chapter 2 might object to this, claiming that the position rests on a fudging of two distinct uses of the word 'good'. To live a good life might mean to live a life that is morally good, in a sense that means doing one's duties to others, or it might mean being successful in self-interested terms. The two need not coincide. I can successfully dominate and exploit others and this might be good for me and bad for them: so they may not think of me as a (morally) 'good' person.

I think it is important to see this egoistic conception of 'doing well' for what it is: a conceptually flawed and profoundly uninspiring version of what it means to live well, rooted in a perverse way of life which no rational person could want for himself or for anyone he cared about. As Aristotle realised, most (if not all) of the properties we have as human subjects are *relational* properties. To know who I am is to know the various relationships I form with those around me: to be a subject is to take interest in that which lies beyond oneself. All activity, including intellectual activity, has an object and the *identity* of the activity is defined with reference to its object. For instance, the activity of a teacher and the activity of a student are one and the same act, considered (as it were) from different angles.[14] Neither one is meaningful without the other. You can no more abstract me from the actions that make me who I am than you can abstract those actions from their objects. For human subjects, *to be* is to be related. It is not clear that it means anything to 'have' any interests simply as an 'ego', abstracted from one's involvement with other things in the world. So it is by no means clear why the whole point of rational life should be the service of this 'ego'. Any credible candidate for a meaningful life will involve making commitments to other things besides one's 'self': commitments for which one would choose, rationally, to sacrifice one's own comforts and even one's own life (given the right circumstances) rather than give up. A person who has managed to live out an entire life without ever making any such commitments has, in a very real sense, never lived and as such is not a model of 'rational self-interest' but an appropriate object for pity and contempt.

So it is not necessary to fudge the two conceptions of 'the good life' distinguished in the egoist's argument: rather, it is necessary to reject one of them altogether. Think of someone that you consider a terrible person, who has 'done well' in conventional terms and therefore believes himself or herself to be 'successful'. Given that you really think this person is a bad person, would you ever seriously wish you *were* that person? If you would, doesn't this suggest that something is going seriously wrong with your own life? It could surely never be 'rational' to want to be a bad person. Nor could we sensibly wish this fate upon anyone we cared for. Wringe (1999, pp. 288–9) considers why we try to bring up our children to be good people. We hope that they will not turn out to be selfish or cruel for their sake, not primarily to protect society or because their behaviour might reflect badly on us; not, even, because we fear they might be punished for their misdeeds (in which case we would simply hope that they did not get caught). Rather, we do not want them to turn out that way simply because we *love* them. Loving them, we want their lives to go well and we know that a person who lives a wicked life does not live a life that goes well. She may 'do very nicely' in materialistic terms, but if she does so at the expense of others she has missed out on what it is to be human and in the only important sense she has not been a 'success'. (This is why parents whose children do 'very well for themselves', by getting highly-paid jobs in areas such as the armaments industry, try so hard to convince themselves that there is really nothing wrong with what their children do. It would be too terrible to admit that your child was profiting from an *evil* trade.)

Analogously, if our children are kind, thoughtful or courageous, we are pleased *for them*. We are not pleased because the social order has another useful servant, nor because their goodness reflects well on us: if we had brought up our children to have character traits which made their lives worse, then this would not in fact reflect well on us. (It would hardly make sense to congratulate a parent for bringing up her children to be the willing dupes of others.) Rather we are pleased because their lives are going well: they are turning into fine humans. All of this suggests that we have a clear sense of 'human flourishing' as the correct view of what it means to do well in life. A moment's intellectual honesty should convince us of this.[15] We should be careful to draw one further logical inference: societies which promote crude materialistic egoism promote a perversion of the human good. Insofar as we are influenced by this concept at all, we have been corrupted. Unequal, divided societies where some suffer so that others may live excessively harm the worst off most directly, but they damage all of us, striking at the heart of our humanity. When you walk past a man who is dying way before his time, because the constant stress and perpetual physical discomfort that attends being hungry and exposed to the elements are gradually breaking him down, something of you dies with him. The more successful you are in forgetting him as you get home, turn on the central heating, eat a good meal and tune into whatever mindless diversions will fill up your evening, the more of you is dead already. The claim, so often sneered at by defenders of the status quo (the most corrupted among us), that we have a common interest in changing such conditions is just clear thinking.

Thus we can break down one final dichotomy: between the value of 'community' and the value of the 'autonomous individual'. In contrast to the autonomous agent of liberal political philosophy, whose interests are in no essential way linked to the well-being of his fellows, the truly rational person is not even capable of emotional detachment from the suffering of those around him. Just as it is nonsensical to speak of a 'moral community' which treats individuals with callousness and arbitrary brutality, so we do violence to the idea of a 'rational individual' by suggesting that such a person can meaningfully lack sympathy for the needs of his fellow creatures. This reinforces the point that the virtue of self-direction is not the licence to head off in any direction which takes one's fancy. A proper understanding of one's condition leads to the recognition of that virtue necessary for the meaningful development and exercise of sympathy and the rational person *could not desire* to avoid developing and exercising sympathy.

To use a word which (because of its proud historical association with a philosophy now considered old hat by the followers of intellectual fashion) will provoke a bout of sneering in those readers infected with the cynicism and indifference which is the malaise of our time, the best label for this virtue is 'solidarity'. One must, in life, attempt to discover ways to associate oneself with the needs and struggles of others. This may prove difficult for a number of reasons. The nature of professional life often quite deliberately is structured to prevent meaningful associations of this sort. As observed in Chapter 4, even trade unions have bought into the so-called 'individualist' ethos, selling themselves to their clients as a form of insurance (some even throwing in such 'incentives' as a union-sponsored credit card and membership of private medical schemes) rather than promoting the unfashionably political idea that we have a collective interest in attempting to bring about a more humane social world.

So there are serious problems facing individuals attempting to exercise the virtues of self-direction and solidarity within the context of a world such as this. We all encounter these difficulties to a greater or lesser extent, but they may seem especially serious for those charged with managing the public services. For such persons, the tensions between living a decent life and surviving in the context of one's working environment can be severe. How might they be better equipped to manage such tensions? What insights can be derived from our discussion of moral education that might help? What of management organisations? Although their contribution to ethical discussion has for the most part been unhelpful (*see* Chapter 4), is there anything they could contribute to producing a better educational environment for their members – assuming there are any individuals within such organisations with the courage and decency to start talking sense? I will attempt to make some tentative comments upon these points in what follows.

Chapter 8

The sort of managers we want and the sort we don't want

The problem with being honest is that when there are no straightforward answers, one has to say so. I know nothing about you, except that you have chosen to read a book called *Ethics, Management and Mythology*. If you have decided to find out what this book has to say for itself by turning to the final pages and have just started reading under the last main heading you could find, then please turn back to Chapter 1 and read it in full, to understand what is wrong with your approach. You cannot hope to join the argument at this stage and take away anything worth having, any more than you can join a long and involved conversation right at the end and hope to make a sensible contribution to it. The book (like any piece of work that purports to be educational) offers you a form of intellectual exercise: its primary value is in the thinking it inspires as you read it, so I am afraid your contribution is indispensable. (The next time you read this paragraph you should have a better understanding as to why this is so.)

If you have gone through the text systematically, as I suggested, then you will realise why, without direct experience of the context of your working life, it would be impertinent and imbecilic for me to attempt to say anything very detailed about how you could do what you do better. There are no formulae for living well. So I can't tell you what they are and anyone who claims to be able to is certainly a charlatan. However, I can hope to influence your attitudes at a very basic level, to affect the perspective and the style of thinking which you bring to every problem you encounter. This is by no means a modest aspiration. In addition, I can support certain sound intuitive reactions you may already have developed. Perhaps you have already read a great deal of the literature on 'management science' and thought to yourself: what has this to do with anything? It's nonsense, isn't it? Well yes, for the most part it is. By this stage you should be better equipped to give expression to those instincts and to defend your own understanding of the world against those who would have you internalise the non-sense. The next time you are told that you should introduce certain practices because they have been scientifically proven to increase quality, reconsider the arguments of Part Two. Or if someone tells you a particular set of policies are 'ethical' because they have been approved by some authoritative group, perhaps even by a panel of 'experts' in the field of 'ethics', you may feel inclined to re-read the arguments of Chapter 6 before you formulate your response.

Generally, when others use appeals to common dogmas or the work of theorists as a stick to hammer home acceptance of the policies and practices they favour, the methods of thinking set out in this book can provide some manner of defence. Sadly, you are increasingly likely to need it. In management, in the health service and elsewhere, dogmatism and formalism are in the ascendancy and good intuitive thinkers are rare on the ground. If the context of your professional life seems to be getting ever more bizarre then this is probably not an indication of mental deterioration on your own part: it is more likely a sign of your persisting sanity, in which case the world needs more people like you – so please don't change to accommodate your environment.

Here's the problem. That is easy enough for me to say, but of course you have to accommodate your environment to some extent if you are to survive within it. If the exercise of thinking clearly causes you to be so frustrated with the irrationality of the working environment that you just want to drop out of it altogether, then nothing good has been achieved. For in that case the most intelligent, reflective thinkers will be eliminated from the system, leaving the most uncritical, least thoughtful persons to determine the organisation of services which are vital to our collective well-being. In which case the situation will never change for the better. As I said, there are no straightforward answers. The comments which follow are not meant to be the final word on anything. The most that I can realistically aim to do is to offer some very general observations on the problem of preserving one's integrity in a corrupt context, which hopefully will advance your thinking on such problems in the context of your own working life. I will also say something about what management organisations should be doing in order to foster better environments, if only to reiterate and expand upon some of the points already made at the end of Chapter 4.

Political philosophy and management: goals versus tactics

It would in some ways be comforting if one could bring oneself to take a thoroughly unreflective stance with regard to one's duties. So many problems would go away if one could say, with Wall (1998, p. 15), that as 'servants of the state' it is our 'public duty' to 'espouse' whatever 'ideology' the ruling political party of the day requires us to 'implement' on its behalf. Unfortunately (or, rather, fortunately) once one has learned the distinction between morality and prudence one cannot unlearn it and one is left instead trying to work out how to reconcile the conflicting claims of each. The government may be my employer and this means that if I consistently do not do what it requires of me it will eventually dismiss me. That will be bad for me (in all the obvious ways) and it is also likely to be ineffective as a form of opposition to its policies, since I will simply be replaced by someone who is willing to comply. It obviously does not follow that it is my 'duty' to internalise its 'ideology' sufficiently to 'implement' it – meaning, please note, to impose it on others. To think that it does is to blur the crucial logical distinction between the goals we should have (the subject matter of moral thinking) and the tactics we should employ to achieve them (the subject matter of prudential thinking). As we shall see, there must be a relationship between the two and in any imperfect world it will not be a straightforward one. Ideally, my moral goals, in conjunction with the available empirical information, would dictate in a clear-cut manner my tactics. However, given the nature of the world as it is, my thinking at the level of tactics will feed back into my thinking about my goals, causing me to modify them: perhaps forcing me to sacrifice some important goals because they are not attainable or because their attainment would lead to other sacrifices which are even less acceptable.

As a rational human subject it is my primary moral duty to think for myself, to exercise the virtues of self-direction and solidarity. Wall notes (op cit) that when managers have acted on their 'public duty' as he sees it, for instance by attempting to impose the 'market ethos' upon clinical and support staff who 'largely opposed' it (a struggle I have described in more detail in Part Two), many of those staff 'felt that managers were not on their side'.[16] Well, they would be right, wouldn't they? Those managers who saw it as their role to stifle opposition to the new 'ethos', and those management theorists who took it upon themselves to become its ideologues, quite obviously did take up a side in a struggle: they took the side of the powerful against a dedicated and conscientious workforce struggling to preserve decent values in their working environment. As I have suggested (Chapter 4), managers should see their moral duties rather differently. Meaningful languages of evaluation can only be constructed by persons with a detailed knowledge of the practices of the area to be evaluated. To talk sense about how one ought to conduct oneself in a given area, one needs detailed contextual knowledge of that area, not training in an ideologically loaded language which abstracts from the specific goals of the area in question. Instead of attempting to communicate the values of the dominant political ethos to the health service, managers should be attempting to listen to workers in the service and engage with them in a *serious* dialogue about how to evaluate practice. They should then attempt to think creatively about how to communicate the needs of the service to the broader social world.

These points are likely to be immediately dismissed as unrealistic. Managers, it will be objected, are as a matter of fact accountable to their employers, which in the context of the NHS means the UK government. To see what is wrong with this objection, it is necessary to consider (briefly) the distinction between social realism (advocated in Chapter 6) and moral realism (advocated in Chapter 7). This distinction is important since without it we cannot have a proper appreciation of the difference between thinking about moral starting points and thinking about tactics.

We must think clearly in order to determine both how the world is and how it ought to be. We must not confuse the two. As we have seen, such a confusion precludes the possibility that there is a radical difference between the way things are and how they should be, consequently loading the ethical dice in favour of the status quo. It embodies the assumption that one can only identify something as wrong if one has some method for changing it which can be fairly easily implemented, given the world as it is. This serves to stifle our sense of moral outrage, since we are encouraged to feel that we are somehow not supposed to get upset about a situation unless we already have in mind some quick fix for it. Yet it is the persistence of a sense of outrage that enables dissatisfaction with what is wrong to grow: only when that sense becomes widespread will genuine social change occur. So fudging this distinction is one way to undermine the motivating force behind any long-term change. Because of this confusion, radical critics of the status quo (from Godwin to Marx) have been represented as having an unrealistic view of social reality. To say that there is much that needs to be changed before we will live in anything resembling a decent society is equated with the claim that the social order is likely to change accordingly within the next few years (or that one has hold of some simple formula to make it so). When it doesn't, apologists for that order will sneer and say that the radical critics have been conclusively refuted.[17]

Bearing this in mind, we can see the error of the objection that my view of the 'duties' of managers is less 'realistic' than Wall's. Of course it will be difficult for individual managers to discover and represent the collective views of the workforce to their superiors and there will be severe limits on their options to express solidarity with that workforce while retaining their position. This does not show that these basic inclinations should not be their moral starting point. The questions about tactics still remain, however. Before saying what little one can say about such questions in a work of theory of this sort, it is worth asking a logically prior question: what sort of moral education is likely to produce managers who have the right moral starting point? This brings us directly to the issue of the sort of managers we want, and the sort we don't want.

Vocational education

At the moment management education, along with vocational education generally, seems to be heading in quite the wrong direction. If vocational education is to be a good thing, then it must represent a partnership between the academic and the practical. It requires doing two quite different sorts of thing at once. Via its 'academic' branch it needs to develop general thinking skills, producing people with sound intellectual instincts to ask the right questions, criticise conceptualisations of practice which are confused, identify the various different types of problem which a situation may present and draw valid inferences from the evidence available. A person so educated can integrate various aspects of experience to find for herself new knowledge in the situations she encounters. In other words, the goal of the academic component of a proper vocational education should be the goal of academic education more generally: it is not to produce better teachers, nurses or managers but rather to produce *people* who are better equipped to fill those roles. As such it should aim to broaden horizons, to equip people with a richer conception of life and practice in the most general terms, encouraging them to think beyond any preconceived notions they may have as to what is 'relevant' to their lives. By being encouraged to think in this way people can bring a wider perspective to the specific problems which confront them. Insofar as this education has a moral component, it should equip people with the courage and confidence to think for themselves, with honesty and compassion. This way they learn not the specifics of a given area but rather the general skills to *make themselves* into good practitioners in the areas they go into. There is no substitute for a proper academic education. Not so long ago people realised this.

However, if an education is to be 'vocational' then it will also need to teach people about the specifics of their chosen vocation. For reasons already explained in some detail, I have serious misgivings about the extent to which this type of information can be communicated in the context of a classroom. Via its 'practical' branch, vocational education needs to supply detailed contextual knowledge concerning the practices its students hope to affect in their working lives. This requires 'hands-on' training. Like the general education which academic study should supply, there is no substitute for this type of immediate, experiential knowledge. Of course, our experiences will be informed by theories and so, of course, we will need to apply our general thinking skills in the context of our practice. The point is that our knowledge of the specifics of concrete situations is only supplied by encountering the reality of those situations in the work context. The old-fashioned idea of practical training is as important as the old-fashioned idea of an academic education.

The problem with much of what now passes for vocational education is that it confuses the roles of theory and practice as characterised above. In order to show that its theoretical components are 'relevant' to practice, theories are taught which attempt to communicate not general thinking skills but bits of alleged 'practical knowledge' which are claimed to be necessary (and sometimes, even, sufficient) to practise well. The result is that certain conceptualisations of practice are effectively taught as dogma, being presented as the definitive view of what the practice is 'really' all about. (So legitimising the claims of the theories taught to be 'relevant' because 'realistic'.) When theorists attempt to make pronouncements on very specific matters of professional practice they overstep the limits of their competence. The result is not a partnership between theory and practice but a peculiar hybrid, a form of 'practical theorising' which is abstract in all the wrong ways (paying insufficient attention to the need for immediate experience of a context) and not abstract in all the ways that good theorising should be: it lacks proper academic rigour and it fails to equip people with the general thinking skills necessary to distance themselves from the conceptualisations which affect how they view their practices, and to comment critically upon them. Indeed, if you question the currently fashionable theories you will be deemed 'out of touch' with 'reality' and thought unfit to practise: dogmatism and intellectual repression are the order of the day. At its worst, this sort of 'education' purports to be able to replace people's contextual knowledge (which is declared to be incomplete, partial and subjective) with a type of 'theoretical knowledge' which can tell them, in advance of experience, what concerns are 'relevant' and what features of the world they should effectively ignore.

We have already seen the worst excesses of this approach to education in 'management science', which replaces theoretical rigour with dogma and claims this is legitimate because of the 'practical' nature of its subject matter – while, simultaneously, encouraging managers to ignore those features of the real world which do not fit in with its theoretical presuppositions. Unfortunately this style of thinking is not restricted to courses in management. In much of what now passes for 'nursing education' and 'nursing theory' the meanings of the terms 'evidence' and 'argument' are defined with reference to what has been published in nursing journals, making the 'body' of 'nursing knowledge' self-substantiating. That is to say, to have any grounds to establish any claim whatsoever, it is both necessary and sufficient to find an article in a recognised nursing journal where the claim has been made. If you try to refute a claim by showing it to be logically self-contradictory or by finding empirical evidence which conclusively refutes it, you are likely to be asked: 'what is your source?'. Unless you can find an accredited article which says the claim is self-contradictory you will be condemned for being 'unscholarly'. (This is no joke. I have seen the comments made by tutors on the essays of nurses who attempt to think for themselves: they condemn them for being 'subjective' and insufficiently 'academic'. On the other hand, mindless acceptance of a claim because it has been published somewhere is encouraged as 'scholarly rigour' – so long as it is properly referenced in the bibliography.)

So what sort of managers do we want? Not people in receipt of the sort of 'vocational education' I have been describing. It is astonishing that the principle that 'there is no substitute for experience' is apparently being abandoned by the very people most inclined to prattle on about how 'practical' they are.[18] To talk sense about a practice one needs to have experience of it. No set of general principles will do instead. If one has never worked in a health service profession then one is in no position to say anything very specific about how to improve the practices of health service professionals. This is why the formalistic approach of management science, with its attempt to deduce specific conclusions about practice in the health service from principles about 'quality management' derived from other areas, could not work. This is also why bioethics had very little of substance to say that could, in any meaningful sense, be 'applied' to the moral problems faced by health professionals. A qualification in 'ethics' cannot enable you to say anything detailed and specific about what practitioners 'should do': philosophy should be equipping people with the reasoning skills to supplement their contextual knowledge so that they can find their own positions on the ethics of their practices – not supplying 'codes' for them to 'follow'. We have neither the right nor the competence to do this.

That is not to say that persons who have been subjected to the wrong sort of 'vocational education' are thereby incapable of functioning well in their chosen professions. Many nurses survive an 'education' in 'nursing theory' and go on to practise well despite it. We all know how they do it: they cynically say the things their tutors want when writing their essays, while learning all the really important things elsewhere. Thus, I do not doubt that there are also people who survive courses in 'Total Quality Management' and nonetheless go on to make intelligent contributions to debates about health services organisation.

However, it would obviously be better if management organisations threw their full weight behind the provision of an education that was actually helpful and stopped supporting forms of education that are in fact unhelpful. If managers are to learn ethics, then it should be taught as a proper academic subject. The discipline of rigorous intellectual thought about the nature of moral existence would be far more valuable an exercise in moral and intellectual development than any amount of idle speculation upon what imaginary people in unconvincingly sketched scenarios 'should do'. Such debates, like the discussions described by Wringe, are more likely to generate a sense of the frivolity and irrelevance of ethical thought than a commitment to decency.

In place of the jargon and dubious principles of 'management science', managers would be better enabled to understand the nature of practical thinking in a social context by being equipped with a basic understanding of epistemology and social science. The abuse of such concepts as 'objectivity' in management literature is shocking, but it only reflects some more general misconceptions about the nature of knowledge, reasoning and value. These misconceptions are not the fault of management theorists: they reflect dogmas that are as deeply embedded in the thinking of a liberal political culture as the contract myth described in Chapter 6. Nonetheless these dogmas affect the thinking of managers and a proper education should enable them to understand and question them. The dominance of the concept of 'value-neutrality' in science has not only held up the advancement of science (particularly social science) – it has also helped to impoverish our thinking about our relationships with one another in very broad terms (Loughlin 1998a). The idea that to be 'rational' one must be 'objective' in a sense that means 'detached', combined with the observation that rational thought is the means for the discovery of knowledge, leads to the view that it is both possible and desirable to understand the world while remaining indifferent to it. This in turn implies that one can know all that one needs to know about one's fellows without ever 'getting involved' with them. Indeed, it gives rise to the belief in the opposition between reason and feelings criticised extensively in this text and consequently to the idea that one should not identify with one's fellows if one is to understand them. (For to be 'involved' would make one 'biased'.) Such a view makes moral education strictly impossible. As I have argued, far from precluding identification with one's fellows, being a rational human subject in the full sense of the word actually requires this. To be 'detached' is not to be 'rational' or to possess 'objective knowledge'. To be at a distance from the concerns and sufferings of others is rather to fail to understand the reality of their lives.

Thus an indispensable component of moral education, for managers and indeed for anyone else, concerns the development of the capacity for *emotional identification* with others. The question for moral educators is not whether this should be attempted but how precisely it should be achieved. Some readers may take offence at my use of examples of real human suffering and the deliberately evocative writing style I have at points employed to illustrate the sheer cruelty and barbarity of certain social processes and the casual violence of our current social system. They may see these illustrations as unacademic asides, excursions into sentiment on the part of a self-indulgent author 'letting off steam'. In fact, they are essential features of the argument: it is the goal of any properly academic project to convey an adequate sense of the reality of the subject matter under discussion. No work can purport to play an educational role unless it achieves this. To discuss the horrors of the world in a 'detached' manner is to fail to convey any such sense and is to distort by default. It is impossible to understand the world while remaining 'neutral' on important questions of value. To be 'value neutral' is to be 'value empty' (Loughlin 1998a, pp. 25–30): it is to refuse to engage one's sensitive capacities or to treat their engagement as a frivolous and inessential exercise. This is to be not 'rational' but blind to those features of the world to which these capacities yield access. If you do not feel then neither do you reason. If managers are to understand the consequences of the decisions they make then they must be able to identify with others, including workers under pressure in the service and worried patients waiting for treatments they may not live to receive. This means that a proper moral education for managers must enable them to engage their imaginative and emotional faculties. This brings us to the most important features of any worthwhile form of education for managers.

It is vital that those who purport to teach management skills should find more effective ways of, firstly, acquainting managers with the reality of practice in the services they hope to manage and, secondly, instilling in them the habit of continually reacquainting themselves with that reality, as it is experienced by the workforce as well as by patients. Ideally, managers will have a background in one of the health professions. Despite the increase in 'specialist management' courses there are many good people working in organisational capacities in the health service who have detailed first-hand experience of the context because they come 'from the ranks': they have demonstrated their ability to manage by first becoming excellent practitioners.[19] Some-times such people are required to prove their fitness to manage by learning some of the silly management jargon we have encountered in Part Two. When they find this ironic, they may fear that by expressing this reaction they will be con-demned as unwilling to learn or as being hostile to 'theory'. Their fears might even be well grounded but if so, this only shows what a bad job their teachers are doing. Proper training will develop their critical skills in order to enrich their experi-ential knowledge. It will not require them to re-describe that knowledge in a language which, intuitively, seems to falsify its nature, by talking about what it means to do well in healthcare as if it meant the same as doing well in commerce or in some other area. For any well-grounded conception they have of what it means to 'do well' in their field of practice comes from their lived experience of the area and their awareness of what is unique to that area. The trick is to get them to reflect more carefully upon that sense of what 'good practice' means which they have *already* developed, to make explicit the knowledge they already have and to think systematically about it. The very last thing training should do is attempt to teach them some new 'objective' or 'scientific' conception of quality, one that suppo-sedly can replace their intuitive or 'subjective' ideas on the subject.

Where a background in a relevant health profession is not in evidence, some form of training which requires immersion in the context is necessary. Any credible management training programme will incorporate a requirement of this sort: the better the programme, the more complete the immersion it will require and the more effectively it will enable management trainees to distance themselves from a management vocabulary when attempting to understand the significance of the practices they encounter. By analogy, most university language courses worth taking still understand the importance of immersion, requiring students to live and work for a period of one year in the country whose language they hope to master. The very best way to learn French is, of course, to come from France in the first place, to grow up in France. The second best way is to go and live in France for as long as possible and (assuming one's first language is English) to be cut off from other English speakers and all that is English for a sustained period of time. As a general rule, those students who manage to find work in the country find it easier to learn to *think* in French than those who attend French universities and are in constant contact with other English speakers during their time away. Just so, those who wish to manage health services well but do not have a background in healthcare must do much more than engage in a dialogue with other workers in the service. They must learn to see the world through their eyes.

As argued in Chapter 7, learning is something we can never afford to stop doing, so education should not be conceived as something one gets over and done with at the beginning of one's career. The second of the two features of good management education mentioned above (acquiring the habit of reacquainting oneself with the reality of the practices one hopes to organise) is therefore the more important of the two. One learns about the experiences of one's colleagues by actually getting to know them. The more distant a manager is from the rest of the workforce, the harder it is for her to manage well. 'Distance' here means social distance: we all know that it is possible for someone to encounter a group of people every day but never see them for what they are, never gain a full sense of what it is like to be them. And without the habit of constant reacquaintance, it is easy to lose sight of what one once knew. (Consider the example of the poor man who becomes Prime Minister, mentioned in Chapter 6: we are easily changed by context, which if we are not careful can wipe away the commitments that used to define who we were.) What matters most, then, is creating environments in which real communication is possible. The hierarchical structure of an organisation is the greatest obstacle to good management and the worst managers are the ones who are perceived, and perceive themselves to be, the 'superiors' of the workforce.

Most managers will claim to agree with this, to treat their fellow workers as peers for whom they have profound respect and to be opposed to the ideas of hierarchy and superiority. You can identify the ones who actually mean it by the way they respond to genuine expressions of dissent and disagreement. Frequently the manager most inclined to appeal to democratic rhetoric will be the first one to pull out the rule book and begin quoting disciplinary procedures when confronted with honest expressions of well thought out opposition to the policies they espouse and legitimate dissatisfaction with the systems they administer. The very structure of the contemporary professional world encourages this: terms like 'line management' directly link the ideas of management and control, implying that the very existence of management requires power imbalances. It does not need to be like this, but a great deal depends on the moral education of managers. As noted above, decisiveness or self-assertiveness should not mean egoism or arrogance. A good manager must display the virtue of humility: if she is to learn how to facilitate good practice then she must be able to learn from others, especially those 'beneath' her in the power structure.

In this respect her attitude must be the very opposite of the ones expressed in some of the appalling documents we have examined in this text, many produced by influential and highly paid managers in the health service. Such managers need urgently to get over the idea that they possess a 'special objectivity' which gives them a 'particular authority' (IHSM 1993, p. 32) because they are removed from the everyday practices of the service, and to learn to view that distance as the central problem to be overcome. Unless they can find ways to think as *part* of the service, to understand it from the perspective of those working within it, they will lack the appropriate form of knowledge to make an intelligent contribution to the debate about how to evaluate it. Equipped with the right attitudes, one can represent the service to the wider social order, rather than functioning as an agent of that order within the service.

Environments in which good practice can flourish

This brings us back to the point about integrity. Even though one has the right moral starting point, the context of management places limits upon the exercise of the key virtues we have identified. There is a conflict between morality and prudence whenever the context of an action means that pursuing the right ends would be tactically unwise. As suggested above, the strategy of preserving one's 'moral purity' by refusing to go into management at all would achieve nothing, except to weed out the people thoughtful enough to be concerned about the moral problems, leaving all the worst people to make the decisions. Many of us (not just managers) have come across situations where we have been obliged to make compromises with what we know to be right because we realise, pragmatically, that our words will not carry the day or because some things are just not allowed by the structures within which we must operate. In such cases, the trick is to know when to fight and when not to fight: to achieve that attribute of the rational character which lies between the extremes of cowardice (the inclination always to give way to the demands of the context) and foolhardiness (the inclination never to give way, which will achieve just as little as cowardice achieves). In short, we need to develop the virtue which Aristotle and Plato alike characterise as 'courage'. For these philosophers, courage is a form of practical wisdom: 'the knowledge of what is to be dreaded and dared' (Plato 1977, p. 61).[20] This requires clarity, sharp reasoning skills, the right moral starting point, and also a great deal of context-specific information, since without that detailed familiarity with the context, you cannot exercise your other skills with the requisite confidence. This is why I began the discussion under this heading by talking about the limits which my lack of knowledge of your specific work context places upon what I can realistically say here.

Two further, general points can, however, be made. Firstly, it is worth noting that the courage to stand up to dogma, to speak on behalf of the needs of the service when these conflict with the dictates of government and/or one's immediate superiors, and the general confidence to challenge dominant assumptions are virtues which can only flourish in the right atmosphere. In many professional contexts, to criticise nonsense, however diplomatically and skilfully, is to imperil one's career. Such environments encourage cynicism and cowardice. At this environmental level, management organisations have a great deal to answer for. It is the responsibility of any organised body with a degree of social 'clout' to do all it can to create the right climate for its members to practise. The point raised in connection with Wringe's argument that since learning is a social process, we cannot teach one value while our institutions embody its opposite, seems very pertinent here. Management organisations seem keen 'to increase the occurrences of pious utterances in the world' rather than to promote real virtue amongst their members. They churn out documents full of talk about empowerment and honest dialogue, while allowing environments breeding fear and dishonesty to continue. It may be an agonisingly slow process, if it happens at all (there may even be problems of the chicken–egg variety), but we need more decent managers and they need to take control of the organisations which purport to represent them, just as the workforce needs to regain control of its supposed representatives in the trade unions.

The second point is related to this: ethics becomes political philosophy when the limits placed on individual action by the world as it is are such as to leave no acceptable answers open. It is of course extremely difficult for individual managers to do very much to represent the service's needs to the wider community, but they should be able to expect a platform within the bodies which presume to speak on their behalf. At present no-one seems willing to kick-start this process, but perhaps things will change.

All of this is quite deliberately general and inconclusive. My point is not to conclude the debate but to leave it open-ended. Indeed, insofar as there has been anything even resembling a debate about the organisation of health services, and of the public services generally, it has not for the most part been a terribly helpful or intelligent one. Certainly it is nowhere near coming to a sensible conclusion. This work is therefore an attempt to start the sensible debate. It is not clear that there can be such a thing as the 'last word' in a discussion such as this, but even if it were possible, no-one is anywhere near formulating that word: certainly I am not. As I have said all along, the only value of what I have to say is its ability to provoke thinking in others. If I can, at least, help even a single reader to think more clearly about these and other practical questions; if I have managed to whet one person's appetite for systematic inquiry into the important questions of life and practice; and if I have helped to arm one sane person in the constant struggle against stupidity that is contemporary social life, then I have achieved my goals. The more of us there are who are prepared to think honestly and critically about our underlying assumptions, the more hope there is for all of us. Let us hope that, if this book is fortunate enough to have a reader such as this, her contribution to the thinking and practice in this area will be substantially greater than my own.

Notes

Part One

1 Some of the arguments of this chapter are rehearsed in Loughlin (2000a, b).

2 As we will see, there is no significant distinction to be drawn between theories of rational decision making and moral theories. Utilitarianism and deontology will be discussed in Chapter 2.

3 There are indeed many other problems with this work. Henry and her fellow contributors purport to employ a range of methodologies, including 'philosophical analysis and synthesis', but the use of such terms within the text is barely intelligible. It is never clear what the authors are trying to achieve, nor how they think they are going to achieve it, and much of what they say is either vacuous or palpable nonsense. The fact that such work gets into print is indicative of a crisis in the academic world and it raises serious questions about much of what passes for 'applied' research and education. I will return to these issues in Part Three. For a fuller review of this particular text, I refer the reader to my review of it, published in *Health-care Analysis* (1996) **4**: 357–8.

4 Have you ever tried to explain to a high-handed administrator from some building over the road why certain 'ideal' solutions or procedures simply have no bearing on your area of work? It is not because you are a bad communicator, nor is it because you are too stupid or too reactionary to comprehend the value of his proposed innovations. Rather, you fail to convince him because he lacks the appropriate knowledge to understand what you are saying.

5 It is sometimes called 'conceptual analysis' or (when applied to moral questions) 'ethical analysis' but 'philosophical analysis' is probably better since not all of the assumptions determining a person's moral stance need be moral in nature. We will see that epistemological assumptions (about the nature of knowledge and about what can be known) and political and social assumptions (about the nature of government and society) can have a major influence on our approach to practice.

6 Oakeshott scholars will notice that I am taking this phrase out of its proper context and appropriating it shamelessly for my own purposes. Well, it's a very nice phrase and it serves my purposes here rather well. He could hardly blame me for being pragmatic. What he says on the nature and importance of a distinctively academic education (ibid, pp. 307–15) does resonate with the points I am making here concerning the need for a 'vantage point' and the acquisition of general intellectual skills.

7 Clearly this is not the idea that Oakeshott means to convey with his use of this image, either.

8 As workers in the health service will realise, this word is frequently a euphemism for 'buggered up'.

9 I recently read an 'account' of a work by David Seedhouse which ignored many pages of detailed critical analysis to report only 'what he was saying', meaning, his conclusions abstracted from his arguments. This 'account' was followed by a series of off-the-cuff responses which revealed that the author really did not understand his arguments: her responses committed her to theories and assumptions which he had refuted in the main body of the text. Sadly, this is typical of the low standard of academic debate found in much of the literature on healthcare today.

10 We are all terribly concerned when a politician 'breaks the rules', but what most people fail to notice is that he almost certainly did far more damage by the rules he upheld or helped to make up. I wrote this section shortly after Peter Mandelson, architect of 'New Labour', resigned 'in disgrace' following a scandal concerning the purchase of his fashionable London home. Apparently it does not strike anyone as disgraceful that a former communist purchases a huge house for £½ million while people with nothing and nowhere to go freeze to death outside. The real scandal, it appears, is that he failed to make full details of the arrangement known to his building society. (He had made his triumphant return to high office, and his second shameful exit, well before the book actually came to print. This time the cause was alleged departure from due process in the case of a rich man's passport application. The lack of a passport deprives millions of poor people of the chance of a decent life: the same due process which killed off his career literally kills thousands of the world's most desperate people – including very many children – every year, as they attempt to flee conditions of unbearable poverty and are driven to utterly reckless measures because of inhuman asylum laws. Needless to say, there have been no ministerial resignations because of these realities.)

11 Humpty (Carroll 1965, p. 174) maintains that his words mean whatever he chooses them to mean, because he is their 'master'. The point, I take it, is that we use words, they don't use us, so we can use them as we please. Carroll allows us to experience Alice's bewilderment at this bizarre conclusion. He might have allowed her the response: 'The real question is, how *well* do you use words: and it is not clear that you can answer this question in any way you please.' Presumably this would have spoiled his fun.

12 This is the important element of truth in the doctrine called 'prescriptivism' (Hare 1983) although we shall see that some of the assumptions defenders of this view made about the nature and limits of philosophy need to be questioned.

13 See, for instance, Nowell-Smith (1965 pp. 140–4), Nagel (1978) and Parfit (1984, part 1). Nowell-Smith gives a more detailed version of the argument sketched in this paragraph, to the effect that egoism makes a claim which is either substantial and false or true but insignificant. Parfit shows that if I have good reason to want to avoid suffering pain in the future, then I also have a good reason not to want other people to suffer: pain is bad no matter whose pain it is. In other sections of the book he questions the concept of the self on which egoism is based. Throughout his arguments are clear and engaging. I would recommend Parfit's book to anyone seriously interested in learning how to think.

14 Parfit (ibid) gives the example of the city of Venice. He does not want the city to sink into the sea and be lost forever. His reason for this is not simply so that he can continue to derive pleasure from its beauty. It is just as important to him that Venice continues to exist after his death, so his reason for wanting it to survive is not 'self-interest', but nor is it the case that his desire is 'irrational'.

15 See, for instance, Berkeley's argument in §IV (Berkeley 1972, pp. 114–15) that 'sensible objects' including 'houses, mountains' and 'rivers' are 'things we perceive by sense' and 'what do we perceive but our own ideas and sensations?' or the claim in §XXIII that if you attempt to think of a tree in the park existing when you are not thinking of it then you contradict yourself (ibid, p. 124) since you are thinking of it.

16 Taken from *The Guardian* supplement, 1 September 1998, pp. 8–9.

17 I hope the reader is familiar with this phrase: it is self-explanatory in any case. For a much more detailed review of postmodernist thinkers, I strongly recommend *Intellectual Impostures* (Sokal and Bricmont 1998). The authors show that postmodernists

consistently appropriate the language of science to affect an intellectual tone, without having any idea of its meaning.

18 Hume (1989, pp. 469–70). Again, I might add 'rightly or wrongly', since there is some debate about what Hume is actually saying here. For an excellent discussion of the crucial passage in Hume, and the related logical issues, see Hudson (1983, pp. 253–65).

19 This point is made effectively by Flew in Hudson (1969, pp. 135–43).

20 This was in keeping with a view of philosophy prevalent at his time of writing, as a discipline either primarily or exclusively concerned with semantics.

21 These points are defended in much more detail in Alison Loughlin's *Alienation and Value-Neutrality* (1998a, pp. 48–62), where they are used to explain the relationship between reason, value and imagination in ethics, science and social theory. I would strongly recommend this work to anyone seeking a readable introduction to these areas.

22 He goes on (ibid, p. 171) effectively to deny that it is possible for anyone to owe anyone else a favour.

23 Godwin's daughter was Mary Shelley, best known for writing the novel *Frankenstein*, and it is not unreasonable to speculate that Godwin's curiously impersonal approach to the ethics of family life may have had some influence on the preconceptions evident in his daughter's work. However, there is evidence that Godwin was not wholly untouched by sentimentality. It seems that in the earliest version of the *Enquiry Concerning Political Justice*, the 'valet' of the example was the Archbishop's 'maid', who might be one's 'sister' or 'mother', but that even the ultra-detached Godwin could not quite bring himself to leave his mum behind, so he changed the example.

24 I owe this illustration to a conversation with a former student of mine at the MMU, Martin Packer.

25 Also, there are many values which seem *incommensurable*, in that the attempt to incorporate them into a utilitarian calculation seems not only difficult but meaningless. Consider the question 'should we allow hundreds of elderly people to suffer conditions which reduce their mobility, diminish their dignity and potentially shorten their lives, in order to offer a 10–15% chance of survival to a relatively small group of very young children with a rare disease?' It is nonsense to develop a calculus into which we can feed these features of reality to find the 'best' answer. However, it is also worth noting that there is no clear answer as to where (in

deontological terms) our 'duties' lie, either. Anyone who thinks there is just fails to appreciate one side of the problem or the other. The implications of this for the debate about 'rationing' are developed in Chapter 6.

26 I mention Prichard and Ross although I only go on to discuss Moore. For a clear critical account of these authors see Hudson (1983, pp. 87–98).

27 Perhaps I have read too much postmodernist philosophy.

28 Those readers who are looking for easy points to criticise, please note: I at no point say that this is *all* we need to make sound judgements. I will say a little more about what else we need in Part Four.

Part Two

1 Some of the arguments of Part Two are rehearsed in Loughlin (1993a, 1994b and 1996). Sections of these articles are reprinted with the permission of the publishers.

2 I owe a debt of gratitude to Dr Edward Harris of Auckland, whose helpful comments on the paper that eventually became this chapter, and whose thoughtful words and enthusiastic support in further correspondence both encouraged me to develop my ideas in this area and helped improve my arguments.

3 Al-Assaf and Schmele (1993, p. 3) claim that quality is in fact one of three 'major cornerstones', the others being 'access' and 'cost', but that these stones constantly 'impact one another' (presumably chipping off several minor cornerstones in the process).

4 Listen carefully to any New Labour mouthpiece talk on almost any issue for any period of time. The style of talking (the perpetual use of linguistic innovation, non-standard grammar and sentences peppered liberally with buzzwords) seems as much part of the uniform as the ultra-smart suit and the Orwellian double-think. Hear the Education Secretary telling teachers they should 'focus on the positive' and learn to 'celebrate' the closure of a school as an 'opportunity to rebuild'. The ability to put together a coherent argument is symptomatic of a failure to be 'on message'. We have almost forgotten what real political oratory sounds like. We have almost forgotten what a real debate sounds like. As Orwell pointed out, the way to control what people think is to first control the way

they talk. The use of gibberish in place of honest and coherent dialogue is a direct attack on our ability to think.

5 I am sure the reader is familiar with this. 'First they came for the Jews, but I did nothing, for I was not a Jew. Then they came for the communists, but I did nothing. . .'

6 Jones and Macilwaine (1991, p. 21) float the idea that lack of quality may be the cause of '40% of operating costs in a service agency', while the slightly more conservative Brooks (1992, p. 19) suggests the figure is 'enormous . . . possibly as high as 35%'. The authors are not in a position to debate their differences, however, since neither article explains how the figure is calculated.

7 It is often claimed that TQM and CQI go hand in hand, but it is not clear to me how one can have achieved 'total' quality and for it also to be possible to go on continually improving quality. Like the word 'quality', the meaning of the word 'total' is unclear in management theory. Its emphatic tone, rather than its semantic content, seems to be the source of its popularity.

8 Note the evangelical tone of this opening comment. The whole enterprise is justified by an unexplained 'conviction' on the part of the DGM, who is here testifying to that conviction: the article does not make it obvious, but if we turn to the last page to read the details of the writers, we see that one of them is the DGM.

9 There is an exception to this general rule. When a term functions to denote a 'simple' or 'basic' property, we either say it is 'indefinable' or that it is only susceptible to 'ostensive definition'. We have already seen an example of this in connection with Moore's 'non-natural properties' (Chapter 2). We will return to this type of 'definition' in Chapter 4. If this is what management theorists think the word 'quality' means then, like Moore, they commit the 'referential fallacy'.

10 As opposed to systems for unsystematic measurement?

11 This seems to call for a joke. Rather than supply one myself, England fans may supply their favourite joke about their least favourite England manager at this point.

12 Consider the article by the *Guardian* journalist Lyn Gardener discussed in Chapter 2.

13 The 'hammer of witches', a 'classic text' of its time on the detection of practitioners of the black arts.

14 This term was coined by Ryle (1983) although his use of it in the context of the mind–body debate has been extensively criticised (cf.

Clark 1997). Ryle claimed that Descartes erroneously deduced substantial conclusions about the mind from the grammatical properties of the word 'mind' and other mental terms. My claim here is that management scientists make a similar error, assuming the word 'quality' names something which can be the object of scientific study.

15 Despite the constant appeal to the language and concepts of Eastern mysticism, Pirsig is as 'all-American' as they come. On the next page (211) his protagonist 'conjures up' a 'vision of a Qualityless world'. Guess what, it's 'Communist Russia' and 'Communist China'. (Clearly Phaedrus had never heard of the Bolshoi ballet.) Given his later arguments that Quality is in fact not just a part of but the whole of reality, it would seem to follow that these places did not really exist.

16 The book came out in the early 1970s, before the 'quality revolution' had produced the 'wide body of knowledge' (Heginbotham 1994) its exponents rely upon today.

17 Pirsig's talk of subtracting Quality 'from a description of the world as we know it' indicates that he has not grasped the distinction between the descriptive and evaluative functions of language.

18 Wall (1994, p. 317) takes my attempts to get him to clarify his thinking as evidence that I am out of touch with what he deems 'the more mundane processes of what is called "real life".'

19 For a fuller discussion of ideology than I can give here, see Loughlin (1998a, pp. 123–73).

20 The effects of treating students as 'consumers' are already becoming evident in the phenomenon of 'grade inflation', which is a huge problem in the US and is now, like so many American social problems, being imported by the UK. If a student/consumer does not like the 'end-product' of the 'transaction' (the mark she has been given) she feels within her rights to complain. (After all, thanks to New Labour, she is now almost certainly paying for her education herself.) Academics are under increasing pressure to 'satisfy' the 'customers'. Point out that the consequences of such behaviour are collectively self-defeating (the degree as such is devalued, which benefits no one) and you risk being accused of being an elitist, a conservative and a socialist all at once!

21 How many health gains do you produce by bandaging somebody's arm? One? Ten? Fifty? Take your pick. If the bandage is too tight, how many gains (if any) do you deduct?

22 I am not simply referring to 'soviet communism' here: capitalism has also wiped out the lifestyles of indigenous peoples all over the world. In South America and Africa, as well as in Eastern Europe, the golden arches which form the 'M' of the 'MacDonald's' symbol are now more readily identified by more persons than the Christian cross (Vidal 1997).

23 He said this in the third of his four-part TV series *The Conservative Party*, first broadcast on BBC 2 in 1997. Clark was interesting because, unlike most commentators, he was honest. He was thought of as a hard-hearted man because the philosophy he espoused is hard-hearted and, unlike so many others who espouse it, he did not try to hide this or dress it up in nonsensical jargon.

24 I can imagine certain of my readers groaning audibly as I introduce this point. If that is your reaction, then turn your critical attention upon that groan and consider what it reveals about the contents of the vessel that produced it.

25 I am parodying part of a famous speech by John F Kennedy: 'ask not what your country can do for you, but what you can do for your country.'

Part Three

1 Some of the arguments of Part Three are rehearsed in Loughlin (1994c, 1998b). Sections are reprinted with the permission of the publishers.

2 See Chapter 4, especially the arguments under the headings 'Ideology and the "swiftly moving tide"' and 'Agents of the market . . .'

3 I am thinking in particular of currently fashionable forms of conventionalism, to be criticised in Part Four.

4 The reader will note that I have deliberately chosen a way to make my point that is (in positivist terms) 'unscientific'. A well-chosen anecdote can, it seems, illustrate a general point quite well.

5 I could not resist a momentary sense of triumph when accused, by an outraged health studies student, of 'blatant right-wing bias' in a lecture on health policy. It reassured me that I had thought my way into the position I was presenting at the time, sufficiently to convey a full sense of its power and to provoke such resistance. The triumphant feeling was short-lived, however, since I also knew

immediately how far my student was from achieving a philosophical perspective. My ability to present the views of great thinkers
on the right with genuine enthusiasm made me, in her eyes, a
'closet capitalist' and the look on her face suggested nothing I could
say thence onwards could ever convince her otherwise. She simply
could not make sense of the idea that one can reject a view while
fully understanding its appeal and she would rather remain ignorant than risk changing her mind. As noted in Chapter 1, philosophy
requires intellectual and moral courage and for those who cannot
take the risk philosophy requires of them, a firmly closed mind
may seem the only defence.

6 I am referring here to some of the 'accidents' (meaning, please note,
consequences the likes of which are entirely foreseen but not
officially 'intended' when one fires missiles into densely populated
cities) of the most recent (at the time of writing) holy wars to be
conducted by the Western powers. The comment about poisoning
the environment refers to NATO's (in *no* sense 'accidental') policy
of using depleted uranium to increase the destructive potential of
its missiles and shells. Depleted uranium comes from radioactive
waste produced for the nuclear industry and as I write it is being
employed in the Balkans, despite its horrific effects being known to
NATO leaders. Since it was deployed in the Gulf War in 1991 the
birth of deformed and cancer-stricken children in Southern Iraq
testifies to the potency and durability of this particular advance in
military technology. (Strangely enough, very few of these children
have appeared on our TV screens or featured in the national
newspapers.)

7 I am here passing over many important technical distinctions
between different theories that could all be labelled in some sense
'irrationalist' or 'subjectivist'. For my present purposes these distinctions are irrelevant, since the intuitive 'pull' of this whole genre
of theory is what I am interested in: it is this 'pull' which makes this
type of approach seem attractive to students *before* they come to
study the details of the various theories on offer.

8 On reflection I seem to have missed something here. It strikes me
as incongruous, in the context of a sentence which mentions 'our
political leaders', to label a group of footballers 'thugs and poseurs'.
It is one thing to attempt physically to intimidate a referee or to
deceive that same referee with a theatrical dive. It requires villainy
of an altogether different magnitude to authorise several thousand
killings while pondering the right expression to wear at the press
conference later on.

9 I can say very little about the category of aesthetic value judgements here. Can we ever have 'good reason' to judge some types of music better than others? To what extent is this a 'mere matter of opinion'? The issue is, at least in part, a question of the extent to which aesthetic judgements resemble the other two types of statement (expressions of taste and moral judgements) and the extent to which they differ from each. In line with what I go on to argue, I would claim it is because music attempts to evoke an emotional response (as opposed to a purely physiological one) that there is a role for rationality in assessing the relative merits of different works of music. I don't just dislike The Prodigy: they really are rubbish.

10 So the executioner reasons that capital punishment cannot be wrong and workers at armaments factories jeer at protestors from the Third World while their union leaders parrot their bosses' lies.

11 The contrast with 'NICE' so obviously invites the label 'Nasty' that one wonders if this was in fact intended.

12 Since there are no official guidelines to tell us who should produce guidelines, the guidelines industry is rather catholic in who it employs: anyone with the confidence to claim 'expertise' will do.

13 Bagpuss fans will recognise the reference here. (Other readers, please ignore this note.) I am sorry if this comparison seems insulting to Professor Yaffle.

14 Of course, some people would call this a 'philosophical' argument, just as some people think 'morality' is all about sex (Chapter 2). Like the word 'quality' discussed in Part Two, one can use it in any number of ways but the point is to use it well: what must it mean if we are to have any reason to discuss it, if we are to employ it effectively in a serious attempt to understand anything.

15 According to some (hopefully exaggerated) reports, a similar fate has befallen French philosophy. Apparently, in some of the more fashionable coffee-shops of Paris, anyone willing to talk at length (and preferably incomprehensibly) on any subject generally considered 'deep', be it the inherent purposelessness of human existence or the distinction (or lack thereof) between fiction and reality, is considered a 'philosopher' and is likely to command a large audience.

16 I have since dismembered it. To extend Wall's somewhat unsavoury metaphor, its remains are displayed in this chapter, pp. 168–70.

17 As one who rejects philosophy, Wall of course refuses even to try

out any other ways of looking at the world than the ones he is used to already.

18 This much has already been explained (Loughlin 1995b) in a detailed response to Wall's first brief rebuttal of what he (wrongly) took to be my position (Wall 1994). Unfortunately, in a subsequent article, Wall chose to ignore this response altogether, characterising my view in the following terms: 'managers are somehow incapable of considering matters ethically' because they are 'unable, Loughlin argues, to understand the basic intellectual concepts that have underpinned ethical debate for thousands of years' (Wall 1998, p. 13). He then offers his stock 'reply' to 'my' view. My earlier point about sticking your fingers in your ears seems depressingly appropriate here.

19 For convenience, let us call the sort of applied ethics I wish to criticise 'bioethics'. This labelling is by no means ideal. For instance, Rollin (1989) and Rachels (1982) were both published as 'studies in bioethics' but I would not wish to criticise these excellent works. The problem is that labels abound in this area and there is no one label I could adopt that has not been used to cover both work that does fall victim to the criticisms of this chapter and work that doesn't.

20 At this point I will simply remind the reader of the question raised earlier, to which we will shortly return: who is the debate *for*? Its role is not to bring any more resources into the service: it provides not relief from suffering but *formal rationales* for specific decisions. Who is in the market for *that* product? Answer number 2 above: politicians and the powerful.

21 The influence of Rawls (1971) is so pervasive that it is harder to find examples of texts which do not exhibit features of Rawls' approach than to point to ones that do. Brock (1993) exemplifies the approach at its best, incorporating Rawlsian assumptions about metaethics and justice in social policy into an overall theory of just healthcare provision. Daniels (1985) and Dworkin (1994) owe a debt to Rawls. Even Williams (1995, p. 223) attempts a justification of his QALY approach to resource allocation in terms of the Rawlsian 'veil of ignorance'. Frequently authors incorporate Rawlsian assumptions without an explicit statement either of the extent of the influence of Rawls or of the highly controversial nature of his theory.

22 The many, evidently sincere, assertions that his views are just sheer common sense made by Williams (1995) provide an excellent illustration of this phenomenon. Unable to think away certain

ideological constraints, Williams is genuinely baffled that anyone can disagree with him.

23 Hegel proposed a dialectical theory of history: conflicts within society give rise to contradictions, problems insoluble within the existing social framework, necessitating social change. He believed his own society to be the 'end of history': the process was over; all contradictions eliminated. Marx adopted Hegel's dialectical account but saw that his own society, riddled with conflict and inequality, could not be the end of history. Such ideas still influence political debate. In 1990 then US President George Bush claimed that the dominance of liberal capitalism marked the 'end of history', the final stage of social evolution. Unsurprisingly he cited neither Hegel nor Marx as influences on his political thinking, which he did well to fit into a busy career of signing warrants to send men to the gas chamber and giving orders to drop firebombs on Iraqi civilians. If he was right, if our present state of barbarity really is the conclusion of human history, then it is a story with a particularly low moral tone.

24 And as my earlier points about the contentiousness of the subject make clear, if they did decide to find out what was right by consulting an 'expert', they would be wrong to do so!

Part Four

1 Thomas Nagel employs a very similar image to convey the sense of one's own mortality in the last chapter of *The View from Nowhere* (Nagel 1986, p. 228).

2 Aristotle (1955). I do not aim to borrow legitimacy from association with a great philosopher here. Unlike certain applied ethicists, who apparently know what the great philosophers such as Aristotle, Hume and Kant would have thought about such issues as age rationing and *in vitro* fertilisation, I do not claim to be doing anything so bizarre as 'applying' Aristotle's theory to issues in contemporary health services management, simply acknowledging an influence on my own thinking about these questions.

3 I owe this phrase to David Bates, who first encouraged me to think about the problems of health management in these terms.

4 This mentality in part explains the popular appeal of 'procedural' approaches to justice in political philosophy: however horrible the

outcomes, if they have come about in the 'right' way they are beyond criticism. Variants of this idea are at work in Hayek (1982), Rawls (1971) and Nozick (1996). For a criticism of the assumptions behind this type of theory see Loughlin (1998a, pp. 1–15 and p. 23, note 6).

5 I fear that 'being in sympathy with' is a non-transitive relation. That is to say, I have no reason from my reading of Wringe to conclude that he would necessarily be in sympathy with much of what I have to say in this book. In particular, I have no grounds to suppose he would support the position in political philosophy which underlies my criticism of management theory and bioethics.

6 Wringe (1998b, p. 279) suggests a Kantian view of morality is in influence but for the reasons I have given, the picture in fact implied is (probably unintentionally) more subjectivist than Kantian.

7 It is frankly amazing that our sanctimonious leaders can lecture the Irish on the 'wholly unacceptable' nature of using violence for political goals while, in the next sound-bite, stridently defending their own intensive bombing campaigns. How much more perplexing it must be for young minds not yet inducted in the 'subtleties' of adult thinking to be told that it is wrong for them to settle their own disputes by resorting to force.

8 They may at some point be *made* explicit, perhaps by becoming enshrined in certain laws or codes.

9 This was Dr Kevorkian, labelled 'Dr Death' by the American media. At the time of his trial, the US President ordered the bombardment of Serbia, killing thousands – including young children who were buried alive and incinerated. Strangely the US media did not think to rename him 'President Death'. I imagine such a labelling policy would make it too hard for them to distinguish any one president from any other.

10 Whether or not much of what goes on in bioethics is a proper application of philosophical methods is debatable (*see* Chapter 6) but for the point being made here to hold good it is only necessary that bioethics is not a branch of sociology, which I take it its exponents would accept.

11 As far as I can tell, the long, unpunctuated, jargon-packed sentence quoted above (from page 10 of her introduction) is not her typical writing style. For much of the time she is very clear. Certain sorts of mindset seem inseparably linked to a distinctive academic 'accent': adopt one and the other suddenly comes naturally.

12 I dare say that feminist social scientists could supply one or two practical examples here.

13 Animal liberationists and environmentalists alike should note that my preoccupation with what it means to be a human subject does not commit me to the unreflective assumption that humans are the only proper objects of moral concern. The good human being is not someone who thinks that non-human animals and their habitats may be destroyed for the sake of our arbitrary whims. Clark (1984) adopts an agent-centred approach to ethics for much of *The Moral Status of Animals*, using it to champion the cause of non-human creation against the excesses of a corrupted humanity.

14 Sorabji (1983, pp. 144–5) discusses the implications of this for the nature of thinking.

15 To make a point so obvious it is positively clichéd: the more one loves in one's life, the more one suffers. If I see my pet as an item of property I shall not suffer so much when she dies: I'll get another. If I see my friends as people I pass time with, I won't be so hurt if they disappoint or desert me: I'll get some more. If I never took the time to get to know my parents, if I view them as people I never really 'bonded' with, then their passing will seem to me to be just part of growing up. So is it 'better' never to know love? Do we decide on the basis of a quasi-scientific calculus 'weighing' love's pleasures against its pains? Such a calculation is neither meaningful nor necessary. We know that love and its attendant pain are part of what it is to live a human life because we have the right sense of the human good – which has little to do with the empty project of maximising one's own satisfactions.

16 I imagine this 'feeling' was exacerbated when, as he goes on to note (op cit), the same managers opted to sack many of the staff in line with the new ethos concerning 'employment practices'.

17 Hence the many crude representations of 'Marxism' which abound, few of which have very much to do with anything Marx actually said. Godwin is no longer sufficiently well known to be subject to widespread misinterpretation, but in his time his views were subject to greater distortions than those of Marx today. He cautioned explicitly against the use of revolutionary violence as a substitute for education to change social consciousness, but this did not stop his critics claiming that the horrors of the French revolution 'proved him wrong'.

18 Part of the problem, I realise, is that many people in business and management have very peculiar ideas about 'real life', which for

them means what happens in board rooms: as if all else were illusory. This is perhaps why some of them do not appreciate the need for knowledge of any other context.

19 I know of few academics who would think it appropriate for a Dean of Faculty to have no academic standing, for such a person would have no real sense of what it meant for an organisation to be a good academic organisation. Similarly people working in healthcare may rightly feel that a person who purports to organise health services must have the right background to know what he is talking about.

20 There is some controversy surrounding the question of whether Plato actually intends us to accept this definition. My own inclination is to believe that he does.

References

Al-Assaf AF and Schmele JA (eds) (1993) *The Textbook of Total Quality in Healthcare.* St Lucie Press, Delray Beach, FL.

Aristotle (trans. Thompson JAK) (1955) *Ethics.* Penguin Books, Harmondsworth.

Ayer AJ (1962) *The Problem of Knowledge.* Penguin Books, Harmondsworth.

Ayer AJ (1987) *Language, Truth and Logic.* Penguin Books, Harmondsworth.

Beauchamp TL and Childress JF (1994) *Principles of Biomedical Ethics.* Oxford University Press, New York.

Berkeley G (1972) *A New Theory of Vision and Other Writings.* JM Dent, London.

Bertens H (1995) *The Idea of the Postmodern – A History.* Routledge, London.

Berwick DM (1993) Continuous improvement as an ideal in health care. In: AF Al-Assaf and JA Schmele (eds) *The Textbook of Total Quality in Healthcare.* St Lucie Press, Delray Beach, FL.

Brock DW (1993) *Life and Death: philosophical essays in biomedical ethics.* Cambridge University Press, Cambridge.

Brooks T (1992) Total Quality Management in the NHS. *Health Services Management* **18**: 17–19.

Callahan J (ed.) *Ethical Issues in Professional Life.* Oxford University Press, Oxford.

Carroll L (ed. Green RL) (1965) *The Works of Lewis Carroll.* Paul Hamlyn Ltd, London.

Chadwick R (1993) Justice in priority setting. In: *Rationing in Action.* BMJ Publishing Group, London.

Chadwick R (1998) Management, ethics and the allocation of resources. In: S Dracopoulou (ed.) *Ethics and Values in Health Care Management.* Routledge, London.

Chambers J (1992) Health gain – is there a need for the centre? *HFA News* **2000**(19): 10–12.

Clark SRL (1984) *The Moral Status of Animals.* Oxford University Press, Oxford.

Clark SRL (1997) What Ryle meant by 'Absurd'. *Cogito* **11**(2): 79–88.

Crosby PB (1979) *Quality is Free: the art of making quality certain.* McGraw-Hill, New York.

Curtis K (1993) Total quality and management philosophies. In: AF Al-Assaf and JA Schmele (eds) *The Textbook of Total Quality in Healthcare.* St Lucie Press, Delray Beach, FL.

Daniels N (1985) *Just Health Care.* Cambridge University Press, Cambridge.

Darbyshire P (1993) Guest editorial: preserving nursing care in a destitute time. *Journal of Advanced Nursing* **18**: 507–8.

Davis FD (1997) Phronesis, clinical reasoning and Pellegrino's philosophy of medicine. *Theoretical Medicine* **18**(1–2): 173–95.

Donagan A (1977) *The Theory of Morality.* University of Chicago Press, London.

Dracopoulou S (ed.) (1998) *Ethics and Values in Health Care Management.* Routledge, London.

Dworkin R (1994) Prudence or rescue? *Fabian Review* **106**(2): 10–14.

Eskin F (1992) Developing public health practitioners for health gain: what needs to be different? *HFA News* **2000**(19): 2–5.

Godfrey C (1992) Investing in health gains: an economic approach. *HFA News* **2000**(19): 6–9.

Godwin W (1985) *Enquiry Concerning Political Justice.* Penguin Books, Harmondsworth.

Goodpaster KE and Sayer SA (eds) (1979) *Ethics and Problems of the 21st Century.* University of Notre Dame Press, Paris.

Griffin R (1993) *The Nature of Fascism.* Routledge, London.

Hare RM (1972) *Freedom and Reason.* Oxford University Press, Oxford.

Hare RM (1983) *The Language of Morals.* Oxford University Press, Oxford.

Hayek FA (1982) *Law, Legislation and Liberty: a new statement of the liberal principles of justice and political economy.* Routledge, London.

Heginbotham C (1994) Management worries. Letter to the editor. *Health Care Analysis* **2**(3): 270.

Henry C (ed.) (1995) *Professional Ethics and Organisational Change in Education and Health Care.* Edward Arnold, London.

Hill T, Russell M, Gill S, Marchment M, Morgan J and Everett T (1990) The quality initiative. In: *Introducing TQM – A Training Manual.* South East Staffs Health Authority.

Hobbes T (1968) *Leviathan.* Penguin Books, Harmondsworth.

Hudson WD (ed.) (1969) *The Is-Ought Question.* Macmillan Press, London.

Hudson WD (1983) *Modern Moral Philosophy.* Macmillan Press, London.

Hume D (1989) *A Treatise of Human Nature.* Clarendon Press, Oxford.

IHSM (1993) *Future Health Care Options, Final Report.* Institute of Health Services Management, London.

Jones T and Macilwaine H (1991) Diagnosing the organisation: one health authority's experience of Total Quality Management. *International Journal of Health Care Quality Assurance* **4**(5): 21–4.

Joss R and Kogan M (1995) *Advancing Quality: Total Quality Management in the National Health Service.* Open University Press, Buckingham.

Kelly PJ and Swift RS (1991) Total quality management – 'getting started'. *International Journal of Health Care Quality Assurance* **4**(5): 26–8.

Klein R (1993) Dimensions of rationing: who should do what? In: *Rationing in Action.* BMJ Publishing Group, London.

Laffel G and Blumenthal D (1993) The case for using industrial quality management science in health care organisations. In: AF Al-Assaf and JA Schmele (eds) *The Textbook of Total Quality in Healthcare.* St Lucie Press, Delray Beach, FL.

Liddle A (1992a) Health gain. Health Gain 92: Proceedings from The Standing Conference, Norwich, 23–24 July.

Liddle A (1992b) Why should general managers be involved with health gain? *HFA News* **2000**(19): 13–15.

Locke J (1967) *Two Treatises of Government.* Cambridge University Press, Cambridge.

Lockwood M (1985) *Moral Dilemmas in Modern Medicine*. Oxford University Press, Oxford.

Loughlin AJ (1998a) *Alienation and Value-Neutrality*. Ashgate Publishing Ltd, Aldershot.

Loughlin M (1993a) The illusion of quality. *Health Care Analysis* **1**(1): 69–73.

Loughlin M (1993b) The strange quest for the health gain. *Health Care Analysis* **1**(2): 165–9.

Loughlin M (1994a) Behind the Wall paper. *Health Care Analysis* **2**(1): 47–53.

Loughlin M (1994b) The poverty of management. *Health Care Analysis* **2**(2): 135–9.

Loughlin M (1994c) The silence of philosophy. *Health Care Analysis* **2**(4): 310–16.

Loughlin M (1995a) Dworkin, Rawls and reality. *Health Care Analysis* **3**(1): 37–43.

Loughlin M (1995b) The Wall paper re-examined. *Health Care Analysis* **3**(2): 127–34.

Loughlin M (1996) The language of quality. *Journal of Evaluation in Clinical Practice* **2**(2): 87–95.

Loughlin M (1998b) Impossible problems. In: S Dracopoulou (ed.) *Ethics and Values in Health Care Management*. Routledge, London.

Loughlin M (2000a) 'Quality' and 'Excellence': meaning versus rhetoric'. In: A Miles (ed.) *NICE, CHI and the NHS Reforms*. BMA, London.

Loughlin M (2000b) On the meaning of 'Applied Philosophy.' *Philosophical Inquiry* **XXII**(3): 17–37.

Loughlin M and Pritchard A (1997) The defeat of reason. *Health Care Analysis* **5**(4): 315–25.

Loughlin M and Pritchard A (1998) Returning to the point: a reply to the 'riposte' of Pilgrim and Rogers. *Health Care Analysis* **6**(1): 72–81.

MacIntyre AC (1981) *After Virtue*. Duckworth, London.

Maslow A (1968) *Toward a Psychology of Being*. Van Nostrand, New York.

Merry M (1993) Total quality management for physicians: translating the new paradigm. In: AF Al-Assaf and JA Schmele (eds) *The*

Textbook of Total Quality in Healthcare. St Lucie Press, Delray Beach, FL.

Miles A, Bentley P, Grey J and Polychronis A (1995) Purchasing quality in clinical practice: what on earth do we mean? *Journal of Evaluation in Clinical Practice* **1**(1): 87–95.

Mill JS (1983) *Utilitarianism.* JM Dent, London.

Moore GE (1903) *Principia Ethica.* Cambridge University Press, Cambridge.

Nagel T (1978) *The Possibility of Altruism.* Princeton University Press, Princeton.

Nagel T (1986) *The View from Nowhere.* Oxford University Press, Oxford.

Nietzsche F (trans. Hollingdale RJ) (1968) *The Twilight of the Idols and the Anti-Christ.* Penguin Books, Harmondsworth.

Nowell-Smith P (1965) *Ethics.* Penguin Books, Harmondsworth.

Nozick R (1996) *Anarchy, State and Utopia.* Blackwell, Oxford.

Oakeshott M (1962) *Rationalism in Politics.* Trinity Press, London.

O'Neill O (1986) *Faces of Hunger.* Allen and Unwin, London.

PA Consulting Group (1989) *How to Take Part in the Quality Revolution: a management guide.* PA Consulting Group, London.

Parfit D (1984) *Reasons and Persons.* Oxford University Press, Oxford.

Paton HJ (1972) *The Moral Law.* Hutchinson, London.

Peters DA (1992) A new look for quality in home care. *Journal of Nursing Administration* **22**(11): 21–6.

Pirsig RM (1988) *Zen and the Art of Motorcycle Maintenance.* Transworld Publishers, London.

Plato (trans. Lamb WRN) (1977) *Laches, Protagoras, Meno, Euthydemus.* Harvard University Press, Cambridge, Mass.

Pritchard HA (1949) *Moral Obligation.* Oxford University Press, Oxford.

Rachels J (1982) *The End of Life: euthanasia and morality.* Oxford University Press, Oxford.

Rawlins M (1999) In pursuit of quality: the National Institute for Clinical Excellence. *Lancet* **353**: 1079–82.

Rawls J (1971) *A Theory of Justice.* Clarendon Press, Oxford.

Reinhart L (1972) *The Dice Man.* Grafton Books, London.

Rollin B (1989) *The Unheeded Cry: animal consciousness, animal pain and science.* Oxford University Press, Oxford.

Ross WD (1939) *Foundations of Ethics.* Oxford University Press, Oxford.

Rousseau JJ (1947) *The Social Contract.* Dent, London.

Ryle G (1983) *The Concept of Mind.* Peregrine Books, Aylesbury.

Sage G (1991) Customers and the NHS. *International Journal of Health Care Quality Assurance* **4**(3): 11–14.

Saint-Exupéry A (1981) *Le Petit Prince.* Heinemann Educational Books, London.

Seedhouse D (1995) The way around health economics' dead end. *Health Care Analysis* **3**(3): 205–20.

Singer P (ed.) (1990) *Applied Ethics.* Oxford University Press, Oxford.

Smart JJC and Williams B (1973) *Utilitarianism: for and against.* Cambridge University Press, London.

Sokal A and Bricmont J (1998) *Intellectual Impostures.* Profile Books, London.

Sorabji S (1983) *Time, Creation and the Continuum.* Duckworth, London.

Spicker S (1993) Going off the dole: a prudential and ethical critique of the healthfare state. *Health Care Analysis* **1**(1): 33–8.

Spiers J (1994) Whose side are you on anyway? Sharpening purchaser leadership – a patient-focused trust perspective. *Health Care Analysis* **2**(3): 187–90.

Stevenson CL (1944) *Ethics and Language.* Methuen, London.

Sumner LW (1981) *Abortion and Moral Theory.* Princeton University Press, Guildford.

Vidal J (1997) *McLibel: burger culture on trial.* MacMillan, London.

Wall A (1989) *Ethics and the Health Services Manager.* King's Fund Publishing Office, London.

Wall A (1993) *Values and the NHS.* IHSM, London.

Wall A (1994) Behind the wallpaper: a rejoinder. *Health Care Analysis* **2**(4): 317–8.

Wall A (1998) Ethics and management – oil and water? In: S Dracopoulou (ed.) *Ethics and Values in Health Care Management.* Routledge, London.

Williams A (1992) Cost-effective analysis: is it ethical? *Journal of Medical Ethics* **18**: 7–11.

Williams A (1995) Economics, QALYs and medical ethics – a health economist's perspective. *Health Care Analysis* **3**(3): 221–6.

Wolff R (1986) Robert Nozick's derivation of the minimal state. In: J Paul (ed.) *Reading Nozick*. Blackwell, Oxford.

Wringe C (1998a) Reasons, rules and virtues in moral education. *Journal of Philosophy of Education* **32**(2): 225–37.

Wringe C (1998b) Reasons, values and community in moral education. *British Journal of Educational Studies* **46**(3): 278–88.

Wringe C (1999) Being good and living well: three attempts to resolve an ambiguity. *Journal of Philosophy of Education* **33**(2): 28.

Index